THINK SKINNY
FEEL FIT

THINK SKINNY
FEEL FIT

7 Steps to Transform Your Emotional Weight and Have an Awesome Life

ALEJANDRO CHABÁN

ATRIA PAPERBACK
New York London Toronto Sydney New Delhi

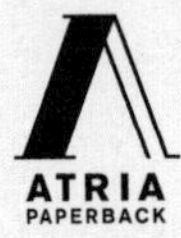

An Imprint of Simon & Schuster, Inc.
1230 Avenue of the Americas
New York, NY 10020

This publication contains the opinions and ideas of its author. It is intended to provide helpful and informative material on the subjects addressed in the publication. It is sold with the understanding that the author and publisher are not engaged in rendering medical, health, or any other kind of personal professional services in the book. The reader should consult his or her medical, health, or other competent professional before adopting any of the suggestions in this book or drawing inferences from it.

The author and publisher specifically disclaim all responsibility for any liability, loss or risk, personal or otherwise, which is incurred as a consequence, directly or indirectly, of the use and application of any of the contents of this book.

First Atria Paperback edition June 2017

ATRIA PAPERBACK and colophon are trademarks of Simon & Schuster, Inc.

For information about special discounts for bulk purchases, please contact Simon & Schuster Special Sales at 1-866-506-1949 or business@simonandschuster.com.

The Simon & Schuster Speakers Bureau can bring authors to your live event. For more information or to book an event, contact the Simon & Schuster Speakers Bureau at 1-866-248-3049 or visit our website at www.simonspeakers.com.

Interior design by Esther Paradelo

Manufactured in the United States of America

10 9 8 7 6 5 4 3 2 1

Library of Congress Cataloging-in-Publication Data

Names: Chabán, Alejandro, 1981– author.
Title: Think skinny, feel fit : 7 steps to transform your emotional weight and have an awesome life / Alejandro Chabán.
Other titles: Dime qué comes y te diré qué sientes. English
Description: First Atria Paperback edition. | New York : Atria Books, 2017.
Identifiers: LCCN 2016050061 (print) | LCCN 2017004109 (ebook) | ISBN 9781501130038 (paperback) | ISBN 9781501130045 (eBook)
Subjects: LCSH: Weight loss. | Food habits—Psychological aspects. Self-care, Health. | BISAC: HEALTH & FITNESS / Healthy Living. | HEALTH & FITNESS / Weight Loss. | SELF-HELP / Personal Growth / Self-Esteem.
Classification: LCC RM222.2 .C4213 2017 (print) | LCC RM222.2 (ebook) | DDC 613.2/5—dc23
LC record available at https://lccn.loc.gov/2016050061

ISBN 978-1-5011-3003-8
ISBN 978-1-5011-3004-5 (ebook)

To every person who, at this very moment,
feels unhappy with who they see in the mirror,
who feels sick in body and spirit, this book is dedicated to you.
Remember that God put us here on earth with a mission.
My mission is to show you how to love yourself and take care
of yourself so that you can one day discover your own mission.
You are valuable, important. You are spectacular and
you have success written all over your future.
Triumph is within your reach.
It's time to love yourself and to take action.
Yes You Can!

CONTENTS

INTRODUCTION

TIME AND AGAIN, I've heard so many people say, "If I lose weight, I'll finally meet someone." "If I lose weight, I won't be depressed anymore." "If I lose weight, I'll have more energy." I myself thought that when I finally lost weight I would find the peace and happiness I yearned for, I'd have friends and would fit in with my peers, and I'd finally receive the love and attention I so desperately desired. But did losing weight fill the void I felt in my life? No. Sure, I did lose 150 pounds, a huge accomplishment, no doubt. But that didn't fix the anger, sadness, and fear inside me. That didn't make friends magically appear in my life. It didn't take away that sense of loneliness that had burdened me for so many years. I had lost the physical weight, but emotionally I still carried a burden.

No matter how hard we try, losing weight without healing our heart and soul, without paying attention to our emotional obesity, without learning to love ourselves, won't fix the underlying problem. The pain remains and that unhealthy relationship we have with food can easily take control of us again. That's why those of us who are chubby—or formerly chubby—gain and lose weight between 10 to 20 times a year, on average. If we don't make a fundamental change from the inside out, if we don't fix the emotional obesity, we will have to live with that up-and-down for the rest of our lives.

I realized the only way to find peace and happiness was to face my fears, confront my reality, identify what was happening to me, and understand where my emotional obesity was rooted. Only then could I learn how to heal my soul.

Some of you might know me from the story of how I lost more than 150 pounds in my youth, which led me to write my first book, *De gordo a galán* (*From Fatty to Hottie*). Others might know me as the host of the top morning show on Univision, *Despierta América*. And still others may have followed *Yes You Can!*, my plan created especially for you, encouraging a healthy lifestyle with a Latin flavor. But few know the deep soul-searching and research I've undertaken to learn everything I want to share with you in this book.

My mission in life is to transform the world. One person at a time, one day at a time, Yes You Can! This has prepared me to give you the best possible information. I've been treated by countless therapists and life coaches, worked with certified nutritionists, and attended an endless number of self-help seminars. I've interviewed dozens of professionals in the fields of health and nutrition. I've dedicated myself to a lifetime of learning, trying to grow as a person, not just to improve my physical well-being but also my mental and emotional well-being. But more importantly, I've actually lived it, in flesh and blood, battling the specter of obesity, bulimia, and anorexia. I know exactly how overweight people feel and I speak from my own experience. In order to change my life, I first had to understand how I became morbidly obese as a young man and why I even let myself get to that point. When I finally understood the answers to these questions, I made the connection between mind, body, and spirit. This had a profound effect on me and caused a total transformation. And that's exactly what I want for you by the time you reach the end of this book.

Patience and perseverance are necessary. But if we don't take the time to look within, deep into our emotions, if we don't take the time to understand what it is we are feeling and why, then we will never be completely healed. Because it's not a matter of simply looking good; we must heal what is inside in order to be healthy on the outside. We are a reflection of our beliefs, emotions, and thoughts.

Everybody talks about nutrition and diet, what to eat and what not to eat, all the latest exercise fads, but no one underlines the importance of feeling good on the inside. No one teaches us that to be truly healthy, we need to work not only on the physical but on the emotional as well. Emotional health is fundamental. And that goes far beyond diet, beyond the visible. It has its roots in the mind. Sure, there are tons of books on dealing with emotions, but none have made the connection to weight gain. None of the books I read spoke to the fat person inside me. None made me feel like they understood my daily struggle to separate food from my emotions, that impulse to want to run to the refrigerator every time I felt anxious or sad or bored or frustrated. And that's why I decided to share my story in detail, expressing the things I'd kept inside about my battle with not just physical obesity but my emotional obesity as well. Because even if you understand the nutritional side, if you don't understand everything you're carrying around inside of you, then your feelings, emotions, and thoughts will remain contaminated. And you will be doomed to a lifetime of unhealthy habits, no matter what diet you choose. Food will control you, instead of the other way around.

I have a friend who underwent gastric bypass surgery and lost physical weight, but it didn't cure the emotional wounds she wore on the inside. She continues to battle the same anxieties that prodded her to eat unhealthy before her surgery. Although the procedure shrunk her stomach, her mind and emotions are still swollen with the pain in her soul. And that prevents her from leading a full and happy life. Many people who manage to lose physical weight but ignore their emotional baggage eventually end up putting the weight back on. Think about it. Maybe that's why your diet hasn't been working. Truly, the mind, body, and spirit are all connected. That's why it's so important to learn to take care of each of these essential parts of ourselves, so that we may be healthy in all aspects of our lives.

No, this book will not magically solve all your problems. It all depends on you, your willpower, your desire to change, and the commitment you make to yourself to heal your spirit. What I'm offering you in these pages are simply the tools to help you on this path. You have my 7 key steps to healing your soul, my personal experience and stories, work guides to help you put your new, personal discoveries into practice, and success stories to inspire you along the way. The power to make these changes, to reach that final step, lies with you—and only you. The fact you're reading this tells me you have the will just within your reach to heal your body and spirit. What are you waiting for? Your moment is NOW!

The most important thing I want you to understand is that for everything to function in your life, you need to heal your emotions first. It took me years to come to this realization, but then again, I didn't have all the proven methods you're holding in your hands. I'm not going to lie to you, change isn't easy. No fundamental change ever is. Yet this is the most important change you can make, for yourself, for your mind, for your soul, for your body, as well as for the loved ones around you. My most sincere hope for you is that you will be able to open your mind and soul wide enough to recognize the darkness of your pain and transform it into light.

If your goal is to lose weight, but you can never manage to stay on track and reach your goal, this book is for you. If you realize that whenever something bad happens in your life, you turn to food for refuge to mask the pain, the agony, the stress, the sadness, or the frustration you're feeling, this book is for you. If you feel like the weight you're carrying around inside your heart won't let you breathe, this book is for you. If you're looking to tone up your body as well as your heart and soul, this book is for you. I want to help you lose that emotional weight so you can feel amazing on the inside, and, once and for all, to look better than you ever have on the outside. I *know* you can do it. Now I need you to believe you can do it, too.

I hope, from the bottom of my heart, that you will see your own experiences reflected in these pages. I hope my story and my 7 steps will help you better understand yourself so you can realize what has been holding you back all this time. I hope you come to understand the pain and fear that have been keeping you from your goals, so you can spread your wings and reach your full potential. And I hope you will make peace with the emotions that led to your emotional weight gain so you can come through this experience physically and emotionally liberated. By opening this book and reading these pages, you're opening the door to a better future and a healthier life. Congratulations! You've taken the first step, and you're right on track.

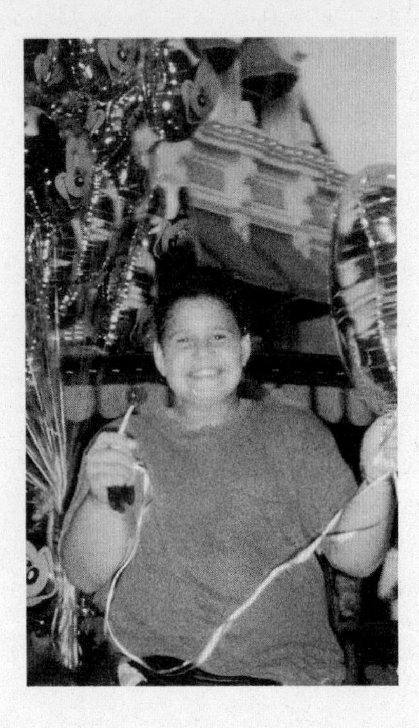

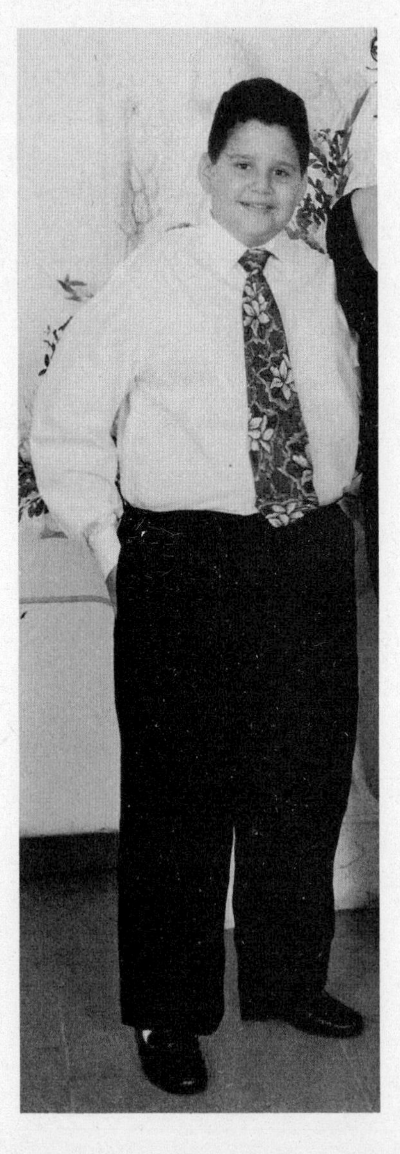

❬ PART ONE ❭

What Is Emotional Weight?

(ONE)

Am I Overweight or Do I Just Think I'm Overweight?

AT SOME POINT, we've all heard the comments: "Oh, he's such a nice guy, but he's let himself go." "She would be so pretty if she just lost some weight." "He's my funny, fat friend." "I don't understand why she let's herself stay that way." These are the labels the world gives us when we're overweight. And boy, do those words sting. It makes us look in the mirror and ask ourselves, "Do I really look that bad? Am I that heavy? Is that all people see?"

In this chapter, I want to discuss a delicate subject for many of us: our waist size. The subject of weight, as you know by this point, is very personal to me. I wasn't born fat. As a boy, I was thin and spritely, but, little by little, I started gaining weight until I reached a critical point during my teenage years. I know what it's like not just to be fat, but to feel like a fat person who will always be a fat person without any hope of ever going back.

But what does it mean to be fat? For some, it's when your clothes are tight or you can't button your pants anymore. When you don't go to the beach because you don't want anyone to see you in your bathing suit. When you fall in love with an outfit at the store but they don't carry it in your size. When you hide when someone wants to take your picture. For others, it's when you can't put your socks on. When it's difficult to walk. When you can't sleep because you have trouble breathing. When your profile picture is just your face because you're ashamed of your body. When getting out of bed, or up from a chair, or climbing a set of stairs becomes a monumental task. We all have a definition. But the common factor is that when we're overweight, we all feel different or uncomfortable. You may come to the conclusion that you are an overweight person, but that's not true. Your body may currently be overweight, but that does not define who you are. It's not something you need to learn to live with. It is a situation you can change.

> *You are not an overweight person.*
> *Your body may currently be overweight,*
> *but that does not define who you are.*
> *It is a situation you can change.*

In my case, as with many people, I didn't realize how much weight I'd gained until I was bordering on obese. And still, I continued to eat and put on more pounds. Sometimes, we don't see the signs of weight gain—or we ignore them. Other times, we just don't have a good measure of what it means to be at a healthy weight. I had no reference point for my ideal weight. I entered puberty in a family that skewed toward the heavy side, one that celebrated kids with big, chubby, pinchable cheeks as being healthy and beautiful.

Both my parents are Venezuelan, but my father is the son of Syrians. So when they got married, my mother had to adapt to his Arab culture, much of which revolves around food. In that culture, a woman shows her husband how much she loves him by feeding him and cooking for him all the time. And my mother took to it right away. That meant that when I came home from school for lunch I sat down to an incredible feast. An average lunch in my house was Arab rice with noodles, tabouleh salad, hummus, pita bread, a plate of marinated olives and pickles, *muchacho en salsa* roast beef, with all the soda and sweetened fresh-squeezed juice you could drink (because sugary drinks taste better). And if that wasn't enough, we never ended a meal before dessert *and* a plate of fruit. Yes, both!

You might be asking yourself, "Wait, isn't Mediterranean food supposed to be healthy?" It can be. But rest assured that a mix of carbohydrates and enormous portions aren't healthy for anyone. Moreover, the only salads I ever ate at home were cabbage with carrots, creamy potato salad, or beet salad. And there was never a shortage of condiments: mayonnaise, sour cream, and cheese. I never saw my mother cook broccoli or Brussels sprouts. The only green that ever showed up on our plate was garnish. For dinner, my mother said she wanted us to eat something "lighter" than at lunch. But that meant a hotdog or a cheese-covered *arepa*, or a ham and cheese sandwich—none of which was actually healthy or "light."

Aside from these daily feasts—which were, to us, simply regular meals—we celebrated every single event with huge spreads of food. From birthdays to graduations, from holidays to new births, each of these special celebrations involved a tableful of lavish dishes. The more food the hosts had to offer, the more it looked like they were taking good care of their family. The dinner table was a reflection of health and prosperity. The same thing went for the kids in the family. The chubbier and more rotund, the stronger and healthier it meant the child was—especially the boys.

In my father's family, each of the boys is named Alejandro, after my grandfather. And when they learned that my father was going to have his own Alejandro to add to the family it was cause for sheer jubilation. For the nine months my mother carried me, the party revolved around her pregnancy. So that's how I came into the world—celebrated and constantly surrounded by these joyous feasts. The party carried on into my childhood. My paternal grandparents made me whatever I wanted to eat, whenever I wanted it. They lavished every delicacy on me. The chubbier I was, the healthier I was in their eyes. My grandmother loved to pinch my cheeks and tell me how strong and healthy I looked, how absolutely perfect I was.

I was gaining way too much weight, but I only ever got positive reinforcement. Without realizing it, they were rewarding me for putting on pounds. What I learned is that this is what it meant to be healthy. Plus, seeing me like that made them happy. They viewed me as a strong, healthy boy who would one day grow into a big, manly man. And my father marveled at how well I ate. I'll get further into that in a later chapter, when we discuss the role emotions play in all this, something I'd learn much later in life.

Given my environment, surrounded by food and praise for being chubby, how was I to guess that my weight gain was anything but positive? Why would I think of myself as fat? When I finally did realize I was overweight, it took me a long time to accept it.

The first time I felt like the fat kid was in the fifth grade. At that time, I had two groups of friends, the Venezuelan kids from school and the Arab kids from the social club where we spent our weekends. At first, when I was just a few pounds overweight, I was considered strong, healthy, and cool. My Arab friends praised me for how big and strong I was. They'd say things like, "You're just like your grandfather," and that made me feel proud and happy. But little by little, this started to change, especially at school. My weight went from being a secondary character to the starring role in my life.

At recess when I'd play baseball with my classmates, it became harder and harder for me to run the bases. As I huffed and puffed, only to be thrown out, I'd hear the others make fun of me. "You got thrown out for being a fat piece of sh—!" Others called me "Cheesy Arepa" or "Shamu" or "Fatty." That's when I started to realize that I was overweight. How could I not? They reminded me of it daily. It only got worse as I got older. At first, I couldn't understand why they were making fun of me. I stated to think, *What's wrong with them?*

Could it be I'm really that *slow and fat?* I had never seen myself that way.

Those first taunts—the first of many in the years to come—opened my eyes and made me understand that my weight wasn't normal, that I was different, that I really was heavier than all the other kids: I really was overweight. It was like flicking on a light in a dark room for the first time. My perspective changed completely. From that moment on, whenever I got dressed to go to school, I was much more aware that my body wasn't like everyone else's. I felt ugly, uncomfortable. I hated seeing myself and realizing I was different because I was fat and they weren't. When I buttoned my pants, I realized the waist was buried beneath something extra, that there was a part of my body that bulged over the top—a great, big belly that had never been so obvious. The elastic waistband or the button left an imprint on my skin. Until that point, I had been used to my clothes always being tight. I'd gotten used to sucking in my gut just to button my pants. I didn't remember what it was like to put on a pair of pants that fit.

This moment of realization filled me with sadness and anger. However, I still didn't quite understand what was happening to me, nor all that lay ahead. At that point, I was about 40 pounds overweight. I hadn't yet become morbidly obese, ballooning to a weight of 314 pounds. I quickly went from being the happy, chubby cool kid, a boy who was always smiling, to feeling different and unhappy. I now saw everything in my life through the lens of this excess burden.

EXCESS BAGGAGE

Being overweight is like carrying around excess baggage twenty-four hours a day, seven days a week. It's like going on an overnight vacation and bringing enough luggage for an entire year. You put on your traveling clothes and shoes, grab your wallet, and then you pack a second pair of shoes and flip-flops in case it's warm. Later, you pack another bag with more clothes because you don't know what to bring, so you pack three T-shirts instead of one, four dresses instead of two, and you keep going until nothing else fits. And then you pack a third bag. You do all of this without even thinking, without realizing you're now going to have to carry all this on your trip. By the time you finally leave the house, you're carrying so many bags that you no longer walk the same. You can barely carry on a conversation because you're huffing and puffing. You can't enjoy the trip or your travel companions because your sole focus is maintaining your balance as you lug around all this extra weight.

Soon, you're carrying around so much stuff that people don't even notice the actual *you* beneath all your baggage. Your eyes, your body, your smile, your personality (yes, even your sexuality), your very essence is buried under all that baggage. It can be isolating, yet it also becomes your refuge. You draw all kinds of attention as you walk by because what do people see but someone waddling along carrying eight bags of luggage? People start to view you as careless and messy. Soon, they begin avoiding you. Now, picture carrying all of that and trying to sit in the middle seat of an airplane or squeezing into a tiny elevator or getting onto a ride at a theme park or simply trying to go out to dinner. It's a constant burden that follows you wherever you go.

> *No one can help you with*
> *all your excess baggage when*
> *you're carrying around an entire closet.*

Think about all those examples. Wouldn't you turn around to get a look at this person who is carrying around so much weight he can't even walk straight? Maybe you'd avoid looking at him instead because it bothers you to see him or because you don't know what you can do to help. Or maybe you just silently judge him and think he must be messy and careless. No one can help you with all this excess baggage when you're carrying around an entire closet. The truth is you're the only one who can help yourself. But it's hard to take that fundamental first step. And with each passing day that you ignore the problem, you bury yourself deeper and deeper beneath this extraordinary weight—a burden that is not only physical but emotional as well.

Over time, you simply come to accept this new way of life to the point where your very essence crumbles and this facade, this baggage you're carrying around, becomes your projection to the rest of the world. Too often, the weight is crushing, but you don't realize it. You can't see yourself from the outside, from behind, from above . . . because you can barely move.

And don't even get me started on how it affects your health. Imagine the effort it takes to move around, the toll it takes on your legs, your arms, your back, your neck, your internal organs, none of which are meant to carry around that much weight. Every morning, you have to get out of bed with all that baggage on top of you, and you no longer feel as agile as you once did. When you go out, to school, to work, to the grocery store, you lumber along much more slowly. Every breath takes effort. Your knees and feet hurt. Your back is killing you. The only thing you want to do is lie on the couch to give your body a break—a body that is screaming out for help while you ignore the signs. Your body just can't handle all the extra bags you keep adding to your load every day. Over time, that pain and exhaustion depress you more and more, sinking you deeper into isolation. You begin to drown in sadness and loneliness, and, defeated, you run to the only thing that soothes you, the only thing that won't scold you or make fun of you, your only consolation: food.

I know this feeling all too well. When I realized I'd become morbidly obese, it felt like there was no turning back. I had no idea how I was going to take all this weight off. I didn't know where to start. Little did I know at the time, I was going to have to address not just the physical baggage but the emotional baggage that started piling on when I was a chubby little boy.

HOW DO I LOSE WEIGHT?

I want to make it clear again that this is no ordinary diet book. I'm not going to give you recipes to help you slim down physically; the advice in this book is about losing the weight that is burdening your soul. To be healthy, you not only have to *look* good. You have to *feel* good. That's the goal in this chapter. I want you to embrace your past, enjoy the present, and let it fill you with anticipation and possibilities for the future. That said, if you're overweight, then having a balanced diet, taking supplements, and establishing a good fitness routine are fundamental to lose weight and maintain a healthy lifestyle.

> *To be healthy, you not only have to* look *good. You have to* feel *good.*

When I finally opened my eyes and realized I was overweight, I tried all kinds of methods to lose the weight. I ate more, I ate less, I stopped eating altogether, but nothing worked. I did all kinds of crazy diets, even the so-called pineapple diet, where I ate a sensible lunch and only pineapple for the rest of the day. But to me that meant I could eat anything with pineapple in it. I would gorge on pineapple cake. If I had come across chocolate-covered pineapple, I'd have inhaled an entire bar of it. That's how my logic worked.

When I was growing up in Maturín, Venezuela, men didn't go on diets. Diets were for girls. That's why I tried to diet on my own, in secret, reading magazines or eavesdropping on the women in the family. At one holiday get-together, I overheard my female cousin say that drinking boiling water helped her burn fat and shrink her stomach. I shudder to think about it today. Insanity! But back then, I was so desperate, I was willing to try anything, including drinking boiling-hot water. In truth, she *did* look thinner, and that only egged me on.

The next morning before I left for school, I hurried downstairs while the rest of the house was still asleep and boiled a pot of water. When it started bubbling, I served myself a glass, took a deep breath, and drank. The pain was so intense I never managed to finish the whole cup, but I drank as much as I could, figuring that the more it hurt, the better it would be at helping me lose weight. When I stepped on the scale on the third day and didn't see a difference, I got frustrated and cast the boiling water regime aside, looking for another magical solution. I would try anything, no matter how dangerous or ridiculous. I went from pineapples to boiling water to the shakes that were all the rage at the time, but I saw no difference at all in my weight. So what did I do? I threw in the towel, figuring there was no hope for me, and I started to eat again. I was depressed and I thought of myself as a hopeless case: *I'm not good at diets. There's no hope for me. It's all in my genes. It's my body. I'm fat and that's all there is to it.*

My real issue was that I was buying into quick, magical solutions, which of course do not exist. I was severely misinformed, I had no idea what a balanced, healthy diet was, and I did not have anyone to guide me. Yet I thought I was doing all the right things. I had even added regular exercise into my life, something that wasn't easy since I was never much into sports or physical fitness. I signed up at a gym and went every day. I started exercising to lose weight; not to achieve a healthy body. All I did were aerobic exercises, but I avoided weights like the plague. I'd heard (incorrectly) that lifting weights would make my body fat harden, and then I would never lose weight. How wrong I was! Weight training isn't the enemy. It doesn't harden fat, but instead tones muscle and helps burn calories. But I didn't know that back then.

I spent years trying different diets, experiencing that frustration at not seeing results, taking note of what worked and what didn't, and trying to understand what made me gain or lose weight. I was tired of eating insipid food that didn't resemble my beloved Latin food. Armed with that information, I started devising a plan that encompassed everything—nutrition, movement, supplements, and emotional health: Yes You Can! (www.YesYouCan.com). I recommend you consult a professional to create a balanced diet and a sustainable exercise plan that will give you results you can see in a mirror (that wicked mirror that can torment us when we're overweight). It's time to turn the mirror into your friend. It's up to you to take that first step.

I want to clear up another thing. There are many types of obesity, such as the kind linked to a disease (such as hyperthyroidism), weight gain due to certain medication, or having a naturally slower metabolism. But in most cases, our excess weight gain is directly tied to our emotions.

Many of us turn to food to cover up our emotions. We eat to fill a void, to forget emotional traumas, or to pacify emotional pain we don't want to endure. But we don't realize that food isn't a cure-all. Yes, it may help you forget your problems momentarily, but that pain, that emptiness, remains. The pleasure you get from food is fleeting; a chocolate bar can't cure your feelings. You can gorge on every delicacy in the world or try every diet known to man, but if you aren't truly honest with yourself, if you don't get to the root of the problem, you'll never achieve the happiness you deserve. I speak from experience. It wasn't until I finally learned to see my emotional weight and its causes that I was able to begin to pursue my dreams.

CAN YOU BE A HAPPY CHUBBY PERSON?

This is a very personal question. I don't know what your experience has been, what you've seen, felt, and suffered throughout your life. I think it's a question each person has to ask him- or herself. So I invite you to ask yourself that question: Is the chubby person inside of you happy? Before you answer, I want you to reflect on your feelings, on your emotions, your heart, your soul, because I want you to answer honestly.

From personal experience, based on my own life and the anecdotes from the thousands of people who have come to Yes You Can! hoping to lose weight, the answer is no, there's no such thing as the happy chubby person. Why do I say that? Because I have lived this and felt it deep in my flesh and bones, and I can say with honesty that I wasn't happy. Every now and then, I might have *felt* happy, but I wasn't truly happy. That image of the happy-go-lucky chubby person is, to me, a mask we put on to cover up our true feelings. It's an excuse we use to avoid confronting the real problem. It's a crutch we rely on to cover up the pain of things like divorce or abuse or loneliness. We act like the happy chubby person to cover up the pain in our hearts and souls.

Nevertheless, when I asked this question on my Facebook page, though many people agreed with me, there were various others who didn't. Many responded that there is such a thing as the happy chubby person. Various men and women defended their point that being chubby didn't affect their level of happiness. And that's a valid feeling because, as I said at the beginning, this is a very personal question intimately tied to our experiences, culture, environment, family, and friends. But what no one can overlook is the topic of physical health. Regardless of how happy you feel, if you're overweight, your body is straining. That's a fact.

A person who is overweight is much more susceptible to illness, and many are already dealing with that fact. And when you have an illness, you can't have true happiness. When your body is overweight, it's a struggle for your arteries, heart, knees, and lungs. Your body is at a disadvantage. It's not functioning the way it should. It's not in balance, and that condition can't be synonymous with happiness.

I don't think the case for physical fitness is debatable, but we have to respect every individual's feelings. Much the same way, we could ask whether you can really be a happy skinny person. The majority might say yes, but certainly not everyone who is skinny is happy. In fact, happiness doesn't have an ideal weight. Happiness can't depend on a scale. It can't be based on a number. It's not about pounds or inches or waist size. Happiness comes from within. We're happy when we figure out our purpose in life, when we're healthy in mind, body, and spirit. When we can face down the pain in our life and finally break free from it.

That's why I want to help you heal your soul, not just your body, so you can discover true happiness. You have no idea how wonderful you'll feel when you understand, accept, and achieve emotional well-being. My hope for you is that you'll discover the true nature of your pain, sadness, and frustration so you can replace them with light, peace, and joy. In this way, you will finally make peace with your past, forgive yourself, accept yourself, and love yourself so you can chase the future that you want.

But first, we need to understand what emotions are, what role they play in our lives, and how they affect our daily life. In the next chapter, let's explore our feelings together so we can begin to understand what's happening with the overweight person inside of us. I want you to stop living in the past, to free yourself from your pain, whatever it is that you are punishing yourself for. I want you to open your eyes and take responsibility for what it is you're feeling *right now*, and, once and for all, get rid of all the excess baggage that's weighing down your body, mind, and soul.

⟨ TWO ⟩

What Are Emotions and How Do They Affect Me?

WHEN YOU THINK of the word "emotions," what comes to mind? Maybe you think of feelings such as joy, sadness, anger, or fear. Or maybe you feel a physical reaction of joy, nostalgia, or rage at a memory. We all have these emotions. We all feel something when we experience something good, frustrating, bitter, or "bad" in our lives. Everyone gets happy when we hear something positive and we all feel frustrated, angry, or scared when we hear something negative. It's part of our daily lives.

However, when we let one of these emotions dictate our lives, when we give free reign to that emotion, that's when a persistent and toxic suffering can begin. From that moment on, that emotion can become a pain that weighs on us. It can become toxic, and, over time, we begin to gain emotional weight. This can eventually lead us to gaining physical weight.

To avoid the domino effect of letting one poisonous emotion topple the rest of our lives, we first have to understand these emotions. Once we identify them, it will be easier to understand if one them has become toxic in our lives.

According to several psychological studies, we have six basic emotions that begin to develop when we're babies. They are:

1. joy
2. sadness
3. fear

4. disgust
5. anger
6. surprise

These are the first, basic emotions we begin to experience in our first year of life. Of course, as we grow, our emotions evolve, and, along with the basic ones, we develop feelings such as stress, worry, frustration, and more. We could make an exhaustive list of everything we feel as adults, but I prefer to focus on the basic emotions, because these affect every aspect of our lives. And they are the basis of all the other emotions we experience.

1. JOY

Joy fills us with hope; it makes us smile; it drives us to fulfill our dreams. It makes us want to live. It's the most rewarding emotion, the one all of us want to experience every day. It keeps us feeling positive, heals our hearts and souls, and gives the gift of well-being. Joy is what we feel when we finally achieve a goal, when we have a positive experience, when someone we like "likes" our photo, when we get that job offer we'd been hoping for, when we can finally buy that thing we wanted, when that song we love comes on the radio and we sing at the top of our lungs. It's what opens the door to happiness in the long run. It's heaven on earth.

However, if we lived in that state all the time, if every second of our lives was sheer joy, we couldn't fully appreciate all the special joyful moments in our life in the same way. They would lose their value. Plus, believe it or not, living in that constant state of ecstasy can become a toxic emotion. There's even a Chinese proverb that explains it perfectly: "Extreme happiness engenders pain." Extreme joy is what we today classify as "mania," an exaggerated manifestation of this basic emotion. During a manic episode of joy, this emotion is no longer tied to any single event. Instead, it bubbles up disconnected to any reason or purpose. It's what can make us feel anxious, unhinged, wound way too tight. And many times, after a manic episode of joy, a person falls into a depressed state.

That extreme joy can also be used to mask other painful emotions. Often we smile and pretend we are happy as to not stir up the pain we're feeling over certain circumstances in our life, to avoid others asking us what's wrong, or to avoid having to address what's at the root of that pain. I know this feeling all too well, because it's what I did when I was overweight. My heart and soul felt heavy. I felt sad and desperate inside, but on the outside, I was the happy-go-lucky chubby guy. I would constantly smile to not worry anyone about my true mental state. That's not a healthy way to be, either. It's important to be honest and share what we're truly feeling in order to identify the problem and overcome it. As we'll explore in these pages, living at extremes can be dangerous. The goal is to keep our emotions in balance. At the end of the day, isn't it amazing to feel a burst of joy after a moment of sadness?

2. SADNESS

No one likes to feel sad, but it's something that happens to all of us at different points in our lives. When a relationship ends. When we're estranged from our family. If we lose our jobs or a loved one. There are a lot of things in our daily lives that can cause us sadness. That's normal. Unfortunately, most of us learn as children to avoid this emotion at all costs. We feel it's not healthy, that we should never be sad. But in reality, it's quite the contrary. Sadness can be good, even necessary.

The problem is that nowadays we've become accustomed to the fantasy that we see on social media, where everyone is always "happy," since no one posts about their failures. We've learned to run from pain and live in a world where only pleasure matters. But that constant pleasure isn't real; it doesn't exist.

And you know what? Being sad every now and then is okay, it's logical, it's normal. It's what brings a healthy balance into our lives. It's part of a healthy emotional state. It helps us to stop and think about what has happened in our lives, to give closure to a chapter. It helps us to learn and grow. Going through a period of sadness helps us to fully appreciate the happier moments in our lives. If we never felt sadness, we could never rejoice in happiness. To know you are happy, you need to know sadness.

Now, like any emotion, taken to the extreme, sadness can be paralyzing. When sadness becomes toxic and takes over our lives, we slip into a depressive state where nothing in life feels worth living for anymore. Extreme sadness robs you of your will to live. You feel like you're carrying the weight of the world on your shoulders. It makes it hard to even get out of bed. It isolates you from your loved ones and can even lead to suicidal thoughts. When this emotion becomes toxic, it becomes something incredibly dangerous, not only to your spirits but to your health. If you feel like you're in a deep, dark hole and can't see the light at the end of the tunnel, seek professional help. If you can't do this alone, turn to someone—a family member, a professional therapist, a friend, a group—who can guide you toward the light you cannot see. You need support and help to keep from drowning within your own tears. Don't be afraid of finding happiness again. You deserve it!

3. FEAR

Fear is primarily a survival emotion. If you're near the edge of a cliff on a mountain, you might naturally feel a fear of falling and take a step back. If you're about to cross the street and see a car coming—and it steps on the gas instead of braking—fear might make you hop back onto the curb to avoid getting hit. When fear is in healthy balance, it's a signal that we're in danger. However, sometimes we develop a fear of things that don't actually present a threat to us. And if we don't become actively conscious of this, fear can easily become a toxic emotion that keeps us from moving ahead in life because we are scared of dangers that don't really exist.

Throughout life, we begin accumulating irrational fears tied to experiences we've endured. These are no longer fears that keep us from truly hazardous situations. For example, if you fell off a horse once and hurt yourself, it's very possible you might never want to ride a horse again. But you can also adopt fears based on what you've seen happen to other people. If you know your cousin got mugged while waiting for a bus, you might become afraid of that stop and avoid it so the same thing doesn't happen to you.

Some people are more afraid than others. But taken to an extreme, fear can become paralyzing. When fear becomes toxic, you might become afraid of things or situations that should never cause this emotion. For example: there are people who fear success, others who are scared of social settings, and there are those who are even afraid to leave their houses. We learn fear as children, when our parents, in their effort to protect us, call out, "Be careful!" Or they yell out a shrill "No!" when we do something wrong and they threaten to punish us. Like all emotions, a healthy dose of fear can bring balance and is essential for survival. But taken to an extreme, it keeps us from growing and exploring new things. No one should live like that. I'm sure you're asking yourself, "Fear as something healthy?" Yes, fear is necessary because it keeps us from painful situations; it is a defense mechanism hardwired into our DNA. It helps us to react instinctively and save us from dangerous situations. It's part of who we are, dating back to the first inhabitants of the Earth. But we have to identify and confront the irrational fears to remove those stones from our path so we can keep moving forward. The only way to combat paralyzing fear is with action. Fear is natural but learning to overcome this fear requires bravery. What awaits you on the other side is something magnificent.

4. DISGUST

Disgust is an emotion that you feel in the moment. It happens when we feel a strong revulsion over something, such as the smell of rotten food or spoiled milk. It's the emotion that protects us from eating something that has gone bad and helps us to survive. It is also what leads us to showering so we don't smell unpleasant. Since it's a fleeting emotion, disgust can't become toxic, but it can open the door to a toxic emotion. If you feel disgust toward everything in your life, sadness or anger can eventually take hold in your heart, which can become extremely toxic.

Let disgust play its role as something that protects you from eating or doing something that will make you sick. But don't let it rule your life and let it keep you from opening the door to pleasurable things that can bring you joy.

5. ANGER

We've all felt anger, irritation, or rage at some point in our lives—probably many times. You experience this emotion when you feel you've been treated unjustly, when you feel misunderstood, when your patience is stretched to the limit, when someone betrays your trust, and in thousands of other situations throughout your life. It's a basic and normal emotion. It helps us defend what is ours, but we have to be very careful with it, because this emotion can easily become toxic.

It's one thing to take a stand against an injustice. It's quite another to be angry every day for no reason. When this emotion becomes toxic, logic and reason go out the window. You feel like you're under attack. You feel like you always have to have your guard up, and when someone comes to talk to you, you respond by yelling. Healthy communication is nonexistent. This not only puts your mental state in danger but also your physical state. Living with anger fills your body with poisonous energy and keeps you in a constant defensive state, thinking everyone and anyone is out to get you. It takes a terrible toll on your mind and body. Plus, the aggression that anger breeds can lead you to say things you regret; you hurt others along the way and that only makes you feel worse. I know this emotion well because I lived through a very aggressive period during my adolescence and into my young adulthood, which pushed me to unimaginable extremes. I'll talk about that in further detail in the next chapter. As with all emotions, a little bit of anger is normal, even necessary, perhaps. But when it gets out of hand, the only solution is to look for the root of the problem and analyze the situation from the outside, which we'll learn how to do in the second half of the book.

6. SURPRISE

Surprise is considered a neutral emotion because it basically gives rise to other emotions, which might bring positive or negative effects. We feel surprise at something unexpected, new, or strange. But think about it: What do you feel when you're surprised? Usually, we feel whatever emotion comes *after* surprise. For example, if you're surprised to learn that you won the lottery, you might then feel joy at knowing all the money you won. Or, you might feel fear at not knowing what you'll do with all that money. If you're surprised to learn a loved one has died, the emotion you'd feel after the initial shock is sadness at the loss or anger at not having been able to do anything to prevent it.

Surprise is more of a gateway emotion that leads you to feel a series of deeper or more painful emotions. It's a passing emotion so it can't become toxic in and of itself because there's not enough time for it to wedge itself into our spirits, not the way joy, sadness, fear, and anger do. That's why when you feel surprised, pay close attention to the emotion you feel immediately after, and make sure it's something that helps, not hurts you. For example, if you've been trying to get pregnant for a long time and then your best friend surprises you with the news that *she's* pregnant, it's normal to feel a range of emotions. Sure, you might feel sadness or frustration, maybe even envy because you haven't yet experienced this miracle from God and she has. But instead of focusing on the negative emotions, be happy for your friend and celebrate that moment with her. Don't let surprises become toxic emotions. Focus on the good. God has a plan. Remind yourself that positive energy attracts more positive energy. Remember the famous quote from the philosopher Michel Eyquem de Montaigne: "I never find myself when I look for myself. I find myself by surprise when I least expect it."

EMOTIONS ON A PHYSICAL LEVEL

Every word, every phrase, every emotion affects each and every fiber of our being. When emotion becomes toxic and takes up residence in our souls, we begin to physically respond to its characteristics. When you feel one of these emotions, stop for a moment and observe what you feel in your body.

That heaviness we feel inside when we're sad, when it reaches its extremes, becomes a heaviness we feel in our entire body. The body wants to rest. It wants to be inert. You don't feel like doing anything; it might even take all your power to get up off the couch or out of bed to walk and stay active. When we feel rage, it has a physical manifestation; we might get red-faced, make a fist and be ready to hit someone from the anger we feel. And that paralyzing fear we feel inside? It might also affect us on the outside, making us cringe and shake like a leaf.

Toxic emotions make us victims of circumstance. For example, sadness is completely natural. But if we let it take control of us and we fall victim to this emotion, it can quickly lead to depression. Say your mom came to visit from another country. When she leaves, you might feel sad for a few days; that's normal. You love her and miss her. However, if this sadness grows and makes you wonder whether she left because of something you did or you torment yourself with thoughts of whether you will ever see her again, you cross over into dangerous territory. You might look to punish yourself and food is often the means for that punishment. We turn to food as a way to resolve this pain when emotions become toxic. But all we do is make it worse.

When we bottle up our feelings or let an emotion take over our lives, we forget about everything else, including our nutrition. We begin to eat without thinking of what we're putting into our bodies and how it may affect us in the short and long run. For example, a woman who was sexually abused might begin to eat thinking, subconsciously, she'll no longer be physically attractive and a target. That sadness she carries around inside—that pain from the abuse—becomes emotional weight, which in turn becomes physical weight.

When emotional pain affects our bodies and we gain weight, we send a clear message to the world around us. Obesity speaks for itself: "I don't value myself. I don't take care of myself. I don't love myself. I don't protect myself." So when we wrap ourselves in this toxic emotion and look for refuge in food, we are actually putting ourselves in danger. We end up even more vulnerable and insecure, and everything becomes harder, more painful. Our mind, body, and spirit become completely unbalanced. We become victims at the hand of obesity and punishing self-loathing. We say, "I'm fat." "I'm worthless." "I'm going to eat as much as I want because nothing matters, anyway. I'm good for nothing, I'm not important and I don't deserve better." Please, I beg you: Stop beating yourself up. You *are* worthy. You *do* have value. You *do* deserve to be healthy. You *do* matter.

EMOTIONS AND BEING OVERWEIGHT CAN TAKE OVER YOUR LIFE

When I was seven and eight years old, my life revolved around school, which I enjoyed. I loved being in school and joined lots of clubs—everything came easy to me. My creative side was just starting to emerge. At a time when boys were running outside to play soccer with their friends, I preferred to spend time in the school theater club. I didn't like sports; the arts were my thing. I joined anything that had to do with acting at school. It was my vocation from an early age.

After school, I'd come home for lunch. That was our family time, and we were close: we enjoyed each other's company, we yelled and laughed like any other normal, happy family. My parents worked tirelessly to give their children all the opportunities they could. When I was young, my father sold grapes out of a van, taught physics at the local university's night school, and, on the weekends, he worked with my uncle at a small shoe store. From seven in the morning to seven at night, he worked at the shoe store before heading over to teach night school, so lunchtime and dinner were the only free time he had to enjoy his family. Those precious two hours, between noon and 2:00 p.m., when my father was home, were sacred.

We'd eat lunch together, and, afterward, as my mother and sisters cleared the table and sat down on the couch to watch their *telenovelas*, my father would take a nap, and I'd cuddle up next to him. That shared hour together was the most wonderful time of the day, because it was my alone time with my dad. At 2:00 p.m., he got up and went back to the shoe store while I stayed in bed a little longer. Around 3:00 p.m., I'd get up and often go to the shoe store to do my homework until around 5:00 or 6:00 p.m. Every now and then, my dad would look over my shoulder to help me with my homework. Okay, that part, I didn't love so much, because when he taught me math, physics, or chemistry, he became The Professor. I'd rather he left me alone to my homework, and I could look up every now and then to watch the business in action.

I'd watch as salesmen came in with suitcases filled with the next season's styles of shoes, and I'd listen to my dad negotiate. Thanks to his hard work and dedication, soon my dad's business grew and he came to own two shoe stores. During those afternoons, I learned a lot about the business world from watching my dad, from how he paid his bills to how he treated his employees. That's where I get my entrepreneurial side. We may not realize it, but everything we witness as children is warehoused in our minds—the good and the bad. That's why it's so important to be aware of what we've experienced in our past: so we can learn from the good and make peace with the bad. Sometimes, something seemingly terrible turns out to be an unexpected blessing.

In the afternoon, after cleaning the house and taking my sisters to their dance classes, my mom would arrive at the business to help my dad. Afterward, she and I would go home to have dinner with my sisters while Dad went off to teach. After dinner, I'd brush my teeth and by 9:00 p.m. I was in bed. That was a typical day for me then—but my life was just about to undergo major changes.

To begin with, in the second grade, the school principal told my parents I should skip a grade because I was doing so well in school. And just like that, I jumped from the second to the fourth grade in one fell swoop. Maybe it had something to do with my dad having taught me my multiplication tables at home. Whatever the case, I soon found myself in the fourth grade, staring down a roomful of new classmates, who were older and bigger. But that didn't faze me. I knew I was at their level intellectually. I was still thin then, and my self-esteem was high. It would be a while before my weight gain dragged down my self-worth.

The teacher told my parents and me that she would try me out for a month. If I couldn't keep up with my classmates, they would send me back to the second grade. That became a huge personal challenge for me: *Oh, you have no idea who you're talking to. There's no way I'm going back to second grade, you'll see.* She'd lit my competitive fire.

I became much harder on myself. At school, we used textbooks named *Resplandor (Brightness)* and each volume corresponded to a particular grade, such as *Brightness* 3, *Brightness* 4, *Brightness* 5 . . . I remember they were huge books. Yet, given the challenge of remaining in the fourth grade, I'd study the book at home on the weekends. That way, I was ready—more than ready—for the material when the time came, and I would not have to suffer the indignity of returning to the second grade. And I did it!

Today, if you ask me why I'm such a perfectionist, so punctual and methodical, I'd say it's because of the time I skipped two grades in school. It required me to focus on my studies, to mature faster, and not only did I stay ahead of the game, I exceeded my own expectations. That period sparked my competitive nature and my desire to do well. But for all those successes, I started to feel a tiny void, a pinprick in my soul that, little by little, grew. An empty space I learned to fill with food.

I think deep down my father realized I needed his presence in my life and he regretted not being able to spend more time with me. So he used those two hours and naptime we had together to praise me any way he could. That's when I realized that if I served myself a second serving of food, he'd turn to me and say, "Look how well he eats! What a champ! He downed two plates already; get him another one so he can grow big and strong and take care of his sisters!" And that's what I wanted, too, to make my father proud. And that's how the approval and attention I so desperately craved from my father became intertwined with food. The more I ate, the more praise was lavished upon me. All right then, I thought: Chow time!

Those lunches were special moments in my life. We had a good time, we talked about our day, and I got the attention

I craved. For his part, I'm sure my dad felt good about being able to give me that time and attention. He must have also noticed that it made me happy to see that he was pleased with me. And so the seduction with food continued. I ate more and more and my father praised each dish I put away, commenting on how big and strong I was getting and how healthy I looked. Of course, we did this all subconsciously. We had no idea of the pattern we were falling into. Neither one of us could have imagined the consequences these seconds and thirds served "with love" would have just a few years later.

Sunday was the only day both my parents were off. Dad would wake up early to clean the displays at the store while the rest of us woke up, got dressed, went for breakfast, and then a walk around town. After a lazy walk, we'd visit my father at the store, and, at about 1:00 p.m., we all ate lunch together at a local Middle Eastern restaurant. We'd sit there talking for an hour or two after lunch and then go for a drive around town in my dad's beige Malibu, listening to his motivational cassettes from Anthony Robbins and Conny Mendez. And of course, we never missed our weekly stop at Cremita, the local ice cream shop. Now that we had fallen into this new pattern, my dad would order me the largest sundae and I, to make him proud, told him, "I want the biggest one!" "That's my boy!" he'd say. "Give him a double scoop!" I'd eat every last bite. After that, it was home to watch a movie on one of Venezuela's two television channels and eat "something light" before going to bed.

Of course, I started gaining weight. Little by little, but unavoidably. To go back to the luggage analogy, if I had to carry a few more bags to spend quality time with my dad, so be it. They would turn out to be heavier than I could ever imagine.

Either no one realized how much weight I was gaining, or no one broached the subject with me, until obesity took over my adolescence. During those years where I slowly gained weight, my family praised my chubby cheeks. They thought I looked healthy, that I was a growing boy, that I looked handsome. I carried more and more "baggage," fueled by all the positive comments, and I didn't realize how much weight I had gained until it was too late.

When sixth-grade graduation came around, I was noticeably heavier. But I barely paid attention to it. I went on with my life as usual. I continued participating in cultural events that would be part of graduation. That year, we performed a play. When they started handing out roles, I was sure I'd land the part of the prince. But, to my surprise, I was chosen to be the narrator. I hadn't yet realized I was too heavy to play any of the other parts. *Okay, so I'll be the narrator,* I thought to myself. At least I got a role. Except there was one more thing: The narrator was a tree. You read that right. I had to dress up like a tree and stand in the corner, narrating for two hours during the whole play. Maybe all of that would have bothered me if it wasn't for the fact I knew my father would be in the audience.

Since my dad worked such long hours and ran his own business, he could rarely make it to any of my plays or school events. But I begged him to hand over his duties for a couple hours and come see me. So he did. I was super happy. My dad was finally going to get to see me in a play, doing what I loved the most—acting. Sure, I was just narrating, but I didn't care. He would be there to see me and that's what mattered. After the play, I ran out excited to see my dad.

"Dad, so what did you think? Did I do well?"

"I didn't see you!" he said.

My heart sank.

"What do you mean?"

"I looked but I didn't see you."

"But . . . I was the tree, Dad . . ."

I'll never forget how crushed I felt that day. My father had finally come to watch me but hadn't seen me. He didn't recognize me because I was hidden behind a couple pieces of cardboard that made up the tree trunk and you could only see my eyes and mouth. He didn't realize it was me. I was so profoundly sad.

By the time my sixth-grade graduation came around, there was no denying how heavy I was. There are a lot of pictures from that day, and not just because it was graduation. I had finished at the top of my class and I was asked to say a few words. But I still had no idea quite how overweight I was. Sure, I'd gotten used to people calling me "Hey, Fatty," as if "Fatty" was my last name. And it was already normal for others to make fun of me during P.E. I accepted my role as the lovable chubby kid and went on my way. Just how fat I'd gotten wouldn't hit me until my first year in middle school.

Until that moment, I'd felt relatively comfortable in my own skin. I'd had the same teachers and classmates all throughout elementary school. And even though they'd started teasing me in the fifth and sixth grade, it still felt like they were just joking around. But when I started the seventh grade, all of that changed. I was in a new grade at a new school, with all new classmates. Plus, I'd started to hit puberty. A kid at that age has a voracious appetite to make up for how fast he is growing, but in my case, things spiraled out of control.

My hope was to come off as cool to my new classmates, but that wasn't in line with the way I looked on the outside. I'd outgrown all the kids' sizes because I was so heavy. So now my mother took me shopping in the men's section, since those clothes were the only ones that fit me. It was tough to have to shop with the adults instead of where all my peers got their cool clothes. *God, I wish the earth would open up and swallow me,* I'd think. I prayed no one I knew would see me shopping there. I didn't want anyone to realize how fat I'd gotten, as if that was even possible. At home, my mother would cut the pant legs almost in half and hem them, so they would fit a child's height. That's how I started the seventh grade: wearing size 38 pants and XL shirts. That's when I started to realize how heavy I'd gotten, although I hadn't yet reached the peak I'd reach a little later.

Back then, I couldn't even see my private parts. My big belly hung over my waist. I had this huge, flabby chest the other kids would soon start calling "bitch tits." During P.E. class, sweat and dirt caked between my rolls of fat. I had dandruff and blackheads, braces on my teeth—and I wore glasses. I started wearing sweaters, thinking they would hide my increasing girth. If you can imagine Miami in the summertime, that's what my hometown of Maturín was like. Now imagine wearing a sweater all day in that weather. I have no idea how I didn't die of heat stroke. So take that all in: the constant sweating from the sweater, the pimples, the glasses, the braces, the dandruff, and all the extra weight. The other kids started calling me the male version of "Ugly Betty."

Still, I had no idea what was happening to me. I wasn't aware of the void inside me that I was trying to fill with food. I had no idea how compartmentalizing that pain was affecting my life. I would learn all this much later. It took a long time. But that's why I'm sharing these deep and very personal struggles, so that you can understand what's happening to you. So you can identify what it is you're feeling and address it once and for all.

PURGE THE TOXIC EMOTIONS FROM YOUR SOUL

Letting a toxic emotion take hold of your heart is like having an uninvited houseguest move in and never leave. At first you're surprised and you can't believe what's happening, and you don't know how to ask them to leave. You're shy and don't want to hurt their feelings, so you just keep your mouth shut. But then you start to feel more and more frustrated because you don't know how to get out of the situation. You hate that they don't offer to do the dishes. You can't watch your favorite shows. But since you're too polite, you swallow your emotions and say nothing. After a while, you may feel your hands tied because you're tired of having this persona non grata in your house but you don't know how to ask them to leave. What's worse, there's a part of us that's gotten *used* to having this person living with us. We might even be scared of what it would be like *not* to have them there. That's exactly what happens with a toxic emotion. It takes up residence inside of us and after a while we don't even know how to live without it. That's what leads to being emotionally overweight.

Now, I want to point out one very important thing. As I said, emotions are always present in our lives. They're part of what makes us human. Our emotions guide us and let us know if we are on the right track or not. We can't shut them off. On the contrary, we have to get in touch with our emotions, listen to them, feel them, learn to manage them, and keep them in balance. They work together to help in our day-to day, but we can't let any one emotion rule our lives.

From my Arab relatives, I learned early on that "real men don't cry." Meanwhile, I grew up in a home with sisters, where the girls had the right to cry, and did all the time. That was normal to me. But if I ever cried, I'd get strict scolding: "Stop that! Men don't cry!" That signaled to me that I wasn't allowed to feel that emotion, that sadness, and I had to turn it off like a light switch. I learned to repress my emotions or hide them. Of course, over time—with the help of countless therapists and psychiatrists, motivational speakers, books, and audio tapes—I've learned that sometimes it's necessary to cry and let out those toxic emotions. Otherwise, those emotions can eat us up inside. Crying can be healing.

We have to know pain so we can enjoy happiness. We have to know darkness in order to know the light. It's part of our path in this world. It's what makes us appreciate the good things in life.

> *We have to know pain*
> *so we can enjoy happiness.*

At the end of the day, all of our emotions help us define who we are and what we believe. We cannot know peace unless we understand anger. How would we ever know the joy of happiness if we've never experienced sadness? And even fear, which can sometimes keep us from moving ahead, can be a signal that we're not on the right track. Everything lies in having balance. And that equilibrium requires daily attention. There will be days when one emotion is out of control. Those moments when one emotion is out of balance are when you have to identify, accept, understand, and learn how to heal. That way, you don't let a momentary lapse turn into a negative force in your life.

The next time you feel pain, sadness, anger, stop for a second to think about where it comes from. Ask yourself, "Why do I feel this way?" Write down your answer so you can start identifying what sets off that feeling. Don't let that emotion turn you into its victim. When you feel pain, don't throw yourself on the bed and ask yourself, "Why me?" Every time that thought passes through your mind, I want you to turn it around and ask the question, "What is the purpose of this pain?" And "What can I learn from this situation?"

Asking "Why me?" looks to the past. It's not about finding solutions. Asking "What is the purpose of this pain?" opens up your mind, triggers new feelings, and allows us to think more intelligently about the subject. By asking "what" instead of "why," you take control of your actions and yourself. Accept reality. Make it yours. Take *responsibility*. It's more useful to ask, "What has this relationship taught me?" than it is to wonder, "Why is it over?" True change happens when you stop waiting and start accepting.

> *True change happens when*
> *you stop waiting and start accepting.*

Asking "what is the purpose of this pain?" is the tool you need to gain the strength to evict that excess emotional baggage from your heart. If you can identify that emotional baggage early on, you don't have to suffer its damaging effects. You can manage it on your own terms. You can say proudly, "I *am* in control."

I allowed my need for attention and approval from my father to take up residence in my soul, and, before I knew it, I'd gone from a slender boy to a morbidly obese adolescent, and it still didn't fill the void. In fact, all I did was make matters worse. That's the story of how I began eating emotionally and gaining weight until it became nothing but sadness and pain. Eventually, the positive feedback I got from my father when I ate wasn't enough because I started craving approval in other areas of my life. It was my new reality when I was being made fun of by my new classmates. As I tried to cover up the deepening sadness with a smile, the happy-go-lucky chubby kid was filling up with rage. My emotional weight had taken over.

⟨ THREE ⟩

Are My Emotions Making Me Fat?

OUR FIRST SOURCE of pleasure after we're born is food. That moment when your mother nourishes you for the first time on your first day of life brings you a tenderness and protection that you immediately associate with your mother's love. From that first moment, food becomes that loving warmth and binds you to this person who brought you into the world. That's why so many of us turn to food when we search for comfort, when we're hungry for human contact, when we need love.

Think about it. Anytime we're hurt, we eat to regain that feeling of being safe. It keeps us company when we feel alone. We are intimately tied to food. This bond is so ubiquitous that it even shows up in our romantic movies. What's the first thing the protagonist does when the guy breaks up with her? She goes right to the freezer, grabs a carton of ice cream, and flops down on the couch to eat it all in one sitting. And she never feels better after. Of course, in a movie, everything gets resolved in two hours. She finds her Prince Charming and her Happy Ending, but in real life, the process can take weeks, even years. And if we keep eating a carton of ice cream every time we feel bad, the only result is that we slowly gain weight until one day our pants don't fit us anymore. Ice cream isn't going to fix your relationship. It isn't going to heal your broken heart.

The problem is, many of us can't separate physical hunger

from emotional hunger—the difference between hunger and appetite. Hunger is your body trying to tell you it needs sustenance. Appetite is psychological; it's rooted in the body's need to feel satisfied. If we're nervous, we eat to placate our anxiety. If we lose our jobs, we eat to calm our fear. If we're broke, we eat to mask the stress. If our friend gets the job we so badly wanted, we eat to satiate that jealousy. However, food exists to nourish us, not to hug or love us.

EMOTIONAL HUNGER

It's worth repeating: Hunger is a physiological phenomenon. It's your body's tool for making sure you eat enough to function and survive. When you feel that emotional hunger, however, that appetite you're feeling is in fact tied to a memory, your mind's bond to a moment of pleasure, peace, happiness, or joy brought to you by that particular mouthful of food. What you're really searching for is to feel safe again. Sometimes we can feel so vulnerable that we turn to food to bring us back to that place where we feel like no one can hurt us.

Emotional hunger leads to emotional weight gain—which ends up as *physical* weight gain. Why? First, because the foods we crave in those moments of crisis aren't necessarily the best for us. You never say, "I broke up with my girlfriend, and now what I really want are some nice steamed vegetables!" You're not thinking about a leafy green salad and baked chicken breasts. What you want, what you crave, what you think you need to quiet the pain is a piece of your favorite pie, a dish of pasta, a big juicy steak with a side of French fries, that candy bar you'd been denying yourself for months. This happens because these are comfort foods. They can trigger neurotransmitters—serotonin, dopamine, adrenaline—in our brain. The body makes serotonin from an amino acid called tryptophan. When we eat sugar, serotonin levels go up because tryptophan triggers the production of insulin. It makes us feel good at first, but only momentarily. Later, our energy crashes and so does our emotional high as we feel regret.

If your boss yells at you at work, you go home and head straight for the refrigerator to quiet that frustration with food. Then what happens? All that sugary and fatty food affects you physically, mentally, and emotionally.

It happens to a lot of us immigrants, too, especially when we arrive in a new country like the United States. Not only do we get saucer eyes at the abundance of food in the supermarket. Not only are we blown away by the portions we're served in this country (and we of course finish every last bite, like our mothers taught us). But we also eat to fill the void of having left our countries, our friends, our families. And that's how we pack on the unwanted pounds little by little. We blame water weight or processed foods or the hormones they use in the meat. But the truth is we're eating so much more than we were before, not only because the portions are bigger or because we're trying new kinds of food they didn't have back in our countries. Rather, we're simply eating more to ease the sadness, the loneliness, the fear of the unknown, or whatever toxic emotion we're feeling at the moment.

If you turn to food every time you encounter a difficult moment in your life, little by little your body becomes accustomed to eating this way. And not only are you going to gain weight, this food that once brought you satisfaction now only makes you feel contempt. It becomes an addiction no different from one to drugs, alcohol, cigarettes, even to your cell phone or Facebook. Vices are habits we feel like we can't control and they can destroy us if we don't stop them in time. A bad habit can become dangerous when it makes us lose control.

If you don't heal the pain inside you and break this vicious cycle with new, healthy habits, you're doomed to keep repeating them. Even if you feel bad about it, you'll wake up the next day and do it all over again, anything to avoid the real problem, which every day only grows bigger and deeper. The key is that we're not paying attention to what it's doing to our bodies, minds, and spirits.

FILLING EMOTIONAL VOIDS WITH FOOD

I know very well what it's like to eat to try to fill a void. And I also know that when it happens, you might not even know what you're doing. If we ignore that void, over time, that action becomes a habit. We never stop to ask what's behind our action; we just simply keep doing it. Nevertheless, our needs and emotions are much more complex than we like to think and they can't be fixed by eating a candy bar or another slice of cake.

According to Louise Hay in her book *Heal Your Body,* obesity represents protection, exaggerated sensitivity, a longing for love. The body is a reflection of our emotions. As you gain weight, your body sends you a clear message: You have a problem you're trying to avoid. You're ignoring the voice inside you that is trying to tell you—through weight gain and illness—that something in your soul isn't right. If you don't listen to it, it only screams louder with heart attacks, diabetes, cancer, and even death.

But if you do pay attention to the warning bells your body is sounding, it can help you discover the roots of your problems, your pain, your sadness or your frustration. Yes, when you finally rip off the bandage and pour hydrogen peroxide over the wound to clean it out, it may hurt at first. But eventually, you'll start to feel better; a peace and lightness will fill your heart, body, and mind with the joy you deserve.

THE EFFECTS OF EMOTIONAL WEIGHT

Weight gain steals life from us. It robs us of experiences. It infringes on our ability to enjoy the present and forces us to live in the past ("I wish I had been thinner") or in the future

("When I lose weight, I'll be happy"). As you struggle to maneuver your body, you start falling behind others. Insecurities arise. You withdraw and begin thinking, "Better I keep my mouth shut before someone insults me; better I mind my own business; better I stay home." Or you might become paranoid. If you go to a gym for the first time and you hear someone laugh, you might say, "They're probably laughing at me." Or "That guy looked at me funny." You start taking everything personally and projecting your insecurities on the people around you. You begin to live in a fantasy world created by your mind and insecurities. You start to limit yourself. You don't even allow yourself to dream anymore.

Over time, we start building up an armor to deal with the insults. In addition to withstanding all of society's judgments, we start criticizing ourselves. We judge and punish ourselves such that we isolate ourselves even further. I found refuge in schoolwork, and when that wasn't enough, I withdrew into solitude. When that didn't work, I became aggressive. Others hide behind denial, depression, excess partying, jokes at their own expense, or a search for constant approval that never arrives. We manage to make everyone happy, except ourselves. We walk our friend to class or our cousin to her appointment or our mother to night school. We do everything not to end up alone, to please others because we don't think we deserve any better. Even when people judge or insult us, we take it to avoid the pain of feeling isolated. We don't trust ourselves. Instead, we only trust in food.

That's where we find comfort and solace. It's where we search for the warmth we so desire. It's the solace we need amid our pain. Because food never yells at us, never judges us, doesn't require anything of us. Food doesn't impose rules. We eat out of boredom or to please others. We eat to celebrate or to drown our worries. We establish a new pattern where, if we don't eat until we feel sick, we don't feel like we've eaten enough. We begin getting used to the pain for that fleeting moment of contentment. That way we avoid the struggle it requires for true and lasting change.

It took years for me to feel legitimate hunger again, the physical sign that our body needs nourishment and not our injured souls. Nowadays, when I cheat on my diet, I immediately feel sick or bloated or gassy and I'm stunned that I could have lived so many years with this being the norm. As a boy I had learned a bad habit, that food was my way of getting attention or receiving love or calming my emotions. I ate because my mother had worked hard to be able to buy our food. Or I ate because my grandmother said things like, "Ale, I spent all this time slaving away in the kitchen and that's all you're going to eat?" I ate because an aunt had brought me a dessert or candy from a trip. I ate because my family was celebrating some event with a huge cake and if I didn't have a slice, they were just going to throw it away. Through it all, I only thought about others but never myself. I never stopped to listen to my own body. I never asked myself, "Wait, let me listen to my stomach. Am I really hungry? Does my body really need sustenance to keep functioning?"

When you fall into the trap of eating without considering the consequences, you'll pound an entree, dessert, and fruit all at lunch and return to work feeling stuffed. You spend the rest of the afternoon slothful and sleepy, and yet, when someone brings a plate of cookies into the office, you'll eat those, too, without thinking about how awful you feel. A few hours later, you go home and eat another big meal, another dessert, maybe a couple of drinks, too, and then go to bed with a belly bursting with food. Yet, it's all you know. You become the victim of your own actions and habits.

You start getting used to thinking that this is how full you're supposed to feel all the time, living on antacids. That's how you drown out your feelings, masking them with massive mouthfuls of food to keep your mind busy instead of having to face any emptiness. You try to deafen yourself to your body's calls for help, but the body keeps crying out. I know how you feel because I've been there. I've suffered through it—for many years. A cookie in your mouth can kill the anxiety for a moment. But it doesn't solve the problem. When you're done chewing, the pain is right there waiting for you.

It's such a powerful and deep-rooted habit that even years after losing all my weight, when I'm sad, frustrated, or insecure, I fall back on my aggressive armor or even find myself opening and closing the refrigerator, looking for something to munch on. The difference is I've learned how to control it because now I understand where that feeling comes from. I talk to myself in the mirror. I say, "What are you feeling right now?" and I write the answer down on a piece of paper. I guarantee you that seeing your answer in black and white allows you to analyze what you're actually feeling at that moment. It opens your eyes to the real reason why you want to eat.

> *You need to . . . find the root of the problem that leads you to eating without thinking . . . to finally find that physical and emotional balance you so deserve.*

When you finally discover why you have been turning to food for refuge—the emotions or feelings you have been trying to avoid—then you can take the next step forward. You need to heal that very deep wound, to find the root of the problem that leads you to eating without thinking of your well-being. And when you find it, you must dig it up, analyze it, and make peace with it to finally find that physical and emotional balance you so deserve.

Nowadays, I rarely turn to food in moments of crisis, but it took time, effort, patience, and perseverance to reach this point. I now understand one has to nourish all areas of one's life, in good times and in bad, to maintain that healthy balance. More than ever, I now realize that to live a happy and healthy life, to lose weight permanently, you have to pay the same amount of attention to your emotions. You have to help your mind "lose weight," by letting go of negative thoughts, destructive beliefs, and painful feelings.

MY EMOTIONAL WEIGHT COMES TO THE SURFACE

It took years for me to discover my emotional weight. When it finally clicked in my head and I realized what had happened to me, I was already much thinner. I had moved from my hometown to Caracas, the capital of Venezuela, and I was following my interest in acting while studying law in college.

As I explained earlier, when I entered puberty, that stage in my life when I wanted to have a closer connection to my dad, I realized that one way to bond with him and get that loving warmth—that protection that I so yearned for—was through food. Every time we sat down to eat, I looked forward to hearing him say things like, "There's the king of the castle! Look at how well he eats!" "Why, you've barely eaten anything. Make yourself a bigger plate!" "Serve the man of the house first!" Those phrases were like applause from my father. It's what my heart was searching for to feel loved. It's what that little boy needed to know that his father was proud of him. I learned that was how I got my father's attention, how I felt loved. *If I want more attention, I should eat more!*

Meanwhile, my mother and grandmother also fed into it. My mother would say, "Hey, do you know how many children are dying of starvation in the world, and you're not even going to finish your plate?" And my grandmother, who loved my chubby cheeks, would proudly say, "I've been cooking since yesterday to make this meal especially for little Alejandro." Even if I was full, I pushed through and finished my plate.

This message I was receiving about my relationship with food started playing a role in other important aspects of my life. At first, I ate for my father's attention and approval. But over time, food became my coping strategy for other toxic emotions that were building up inside me. The more abuse I took at school, the more alone I felt, the more often I felt rejected, the more I turned to the warmth and protection that food provided. But no one ever tells you how gaining weight will affect your life, not just physically, but emotionally.

Of course, as I gained weight, the harassment at school only got worse. The taunts felt like stab wounds on my soul. For a kid who used to love studying, going to school became a daily torture. My new classmates in my freshman year of high school didn't help.

Just walking to class meant enduring a raining down of insults: "Shamu!" "Killer whale!" "Meatball with legs!" To deal with the insults, my first reaction was to laugh. *Either I laugh or I get angry*, I thought. *And if I get angry and get in a fight, I'll end up in the principal's office and they'll call my dad. I don't want my parents to worry because they already work so hard.*

Although I was laughing on the outside, inside I was falling to pieces. It was such a trying and difficult time that I think about it to this day. You carry these scars with you forever. But if you don't heal the wounds in time, they will cause you pain—and hunger—forever. Sure, I was the happy-go-lucky fat kid around them at school. But when I got home, I shut myself in my room and felt so sad and alone that I'd cry and shout at God. Between sobs I'd ask Him, "Why did You make me this way, God? Why me?" Why did I have to have terrible acne and braces and glasses? Why couldn't I be like the good-looking kids in my class? Why didn't any girls like me? Why didn't anyone want to hang out with me? Why did I have to be *fat?* I couldn't understand why they excluded me, why I never got a birthday party invite—the party that everyone would be talking about on Monday morning. Still, I always held out hope for an invitation. All of it isolated me further from the rest of the world.

And let's not even talk about physical education class! What an unholy nightmare! I think those really were the worst days of my life. I had to wear sweatpants that, despite being XXL, were still stretched tight over my body. Worse, it said "Speedo" along the back. The kids would laugh and say, "Look, Chabán's says Speeeeeeeeeeeeedo!" Plus, I sweat when I am nervous so I started wearing an undershirt, but that only made me sweat more. Oh, and not to mention the sweater I wore, thinking it made me look slimmer. I perspired through every layer until there were dark, wet circles under my armpits. The other kids said it looked like I had a pair of *arepas* under my arms.

I suffered so much in that class that I'd make up illnesses to try to get out of it at all costs. One day I'd say I felt like throwing up. Another, that I had low blood pressure. Anything to get out. One day I actually fell and had to be taken to the hospital. My foot hurt when the doctor examined it, but I yelled like it hurt three times as bad, hoping he'd put a cast on it so I could get out of gym class. I figured, *If they put a cast on me, that's three months out of gym class versus one if they just put a bandage on it.* I preferred to put up with the discomfort of a hot, itchy cast and crutches—which were not easy to get around on, being 300 pounds—than having to put up with the insults in gym class such as, "Bounce, Chabán, bounce!" and "It's easier to jump over Chabán than to walk around him."

I was well aware of every physical imperfection by that point: stretch marks, cellulite, spots of discoloration around my neck and armpits, the rolls of fat. My thighs rubbed together and my inner pant legs would always wear out even though they were new. My mom, to save money, would patch the holes so I could keep wearing them a while longer. The sleeves of my uniform shirt had a pair of dolphins on them, but my classmates teased me that mine should be whales instead.

It got harder and harder to do anything. Putting my socks on in the morning to go to school became a feat. It was almost impossible to bend over to tie my shoes. And as I got ready, I started thinking about what they would say about my shirt, my pants, my excessive sweating, my hair, my glasses, the blackheads on my nose.

And don't think it was just my classmates I had to put up with. The teachers were bullies, too. Try as I might in gym class, I always came in in last place and the teacher would underline it by saying things like, "C'mon, Chabán, you look like you're running in slow motion" in front of the other students. Everyone laughed while I sweated and panted.

As groups of friends started to emerge, and since I was a studious "nerd," I tried to use that to my advantage, by saying that I could help with their schoolwork. But they never really became my friends; it was just a business transaction. That never got me invites to go out or to a party. But at least I got to spend a few minutes with other people and I thought I should just be happy about that.

To make things worse, no one in my neighborhood understood I was being "bullied." It wasn't a well-established term. People just thought it was kids' stuff; no one realized then the damage it did to the target of the bullying. No one even talked about it. So of course it never occurred to me to tell my parents what was happening to me at school. Plus, they were already so stressed at work to make sure we had better lives. It seemed wrong to bother them with this silliness. So I just kept it inside and locked myself in my room to cry.

The truth is that besides not wanting to worry my parents, I also feared that they would say something to the principal. Then, she would say something to the teacher and the teacher would reprimand the other students. That would make me the fat class tattletale and would give them even more reason to make fun of me. I preferred to suffer in silence. My only consolation was food.

That's how a sweet and quiet boy put on his armor and became an angry and defensive soul. Anger started to build inside and it eventually erupted into rage, like a volcano. Since this anger was new to me and not part of my temperament, I'd never learned how to fistfight. So I learned to express my anger with my words—and those became my daggers. I'd use them to defend myself.

By this point, everything bothered me; everything irritated me. When my mother knocked on my bedroom door to tell me something, I yelled horrible things so she would leave me alone. I started being mean to my sisters. I'd transformed into a bitter young man, and I'd isolate myself further by locking myself in my room. My parents were surprised, but they attributed this change to puberty, not to my weight gain.

These volcanic eruptions became more commonplace. By the time I was thirteen years old, my aggressiveness became a battle with the rest of the world. I hated everyone and everything. I looked at my parents, who were a normal weight, and my sisters who were thin, and I felt even more alone. I was angry at life, didn't understand why this had to happen to me. I simply couldn't make sense of why God was punishing me this way.

That rage spilled over not just at home but at school. Instead of going after my classmates, I attacked my teachers. I told one teacher, "Yuck, you need to brush your teeth. Your breath stinks." I made another one cry in class, in front of my classmates. I'd become the overweight rebel; I thought that would get me in with the cool kids. But in reality, I was as alone as ever. Even I became a victim of my own aggression. I'd tell myself every day, "You're no good. You're ugly. You're disgusting. You're worthless. You smell. No one loves you. You don't deserved anything good." Instead of protecting me, my aggression was only hurting others and me.

Before I knew it, I'd become the kind of bully I hated so much. Those five minutes I made fun of a teacher were five minutes a classmate wasn't making fun of me. At least in those five minutes, I thought, they were with me instead of against me. I felt like I belonged. In those five minutes, I erupted with the rage I had inside me and no one was attacking me instead.

My aggressiveness and sadness were so near the surface that if I were walking down the street and someone laughed, I'd immediately get in their face and say, "Why are you laughing at me, huh?" I took everything personally, even when it had nothing to do with me. It felt like the world was against me. If I had to go to a family get together with my parents, that happy occasion became my nightmare. I'd spend hours thinking about what I could wear that fit. I'd try on a pair of pants, lay down on my bed to try to close them, and instead they would rip. I'd try on another and another, and nothing fit. Eventually, I'd give up and stay home by myself.

I became more and more isolated. During the last six months of my obesity, I even started waking up in the middle of the night to eat. My addiction to food was so strong, and my self-destruction so complete, that I no longer had any love for myself. I had accepted I was a fat person and yet the more I ate, the more depressed I felt and the less energy I had. *I'm fat and disgusting. No one loves me, I smell, and they let me know it. What's the point in fighting it?* With that mind-set, I threw in the towel and accepted my new identity. I saw no way out and had no hope. I'd cried so many times, had cursed at God so often, that I'd given up. I thought this would be my life. "I'm fat," that was my destiny.

During all this pain, anguish, and hopelessness, I'd think, *Why even live? My life is worthless. I'd rather die and stop being such a nuisance to everyone around me.* My life had no meaning. I imagined my suicide would be a great comfort. I would no longer be a bother, a worthless lump that was only good for insulting. After all, I was the only one in my living hell. I hated myself so much, had so many insecurities, such low self-esteem. The only thing that kept me from carrying out my death wish was my parents and sisters. As much as I wanted to shed this physical and emotional weight once and for all, I couldn't imagine not seeing them again. I didn't want to cause them pain. So I had no choice but to forge ahead as best I could.

I continued to drag myself through life, thinking I had no other alternative, that this would be my life forever. I saw no going back. My problem was that I hadn't yet taken the first step toward making any major change: I hadn't made a commitment to myself. Without that pledge, I'd never accomplish anything.

⟨ PART TWO ⟩

The 7 Steps to Losing Your Emotional Weight

Prepare to Begin Your Life-Changing Transformation

When your emotional weight gain reaches the point that you question whether life is even worth living, it's the red flag accompanied by warning sirens indicating that it's time to get help. Please, don't ignore it! You are not alone. I promise you, everything has a solution. It only requires effort and commitment on your part. I know what it's like to feel such anguish, loneliness, and desperation that death seems like the only option. I know what it feels like to lose hope, to lack goals and dreams. But I also know what it feels like when you can finally see the light at the end of the tunnel. When you finally climb out from the bottom of that deep, dark well and are able to take a step forward. It's not easy, but it is possible. Yes, you can!

I want to make one thing clear: Many of us carry around emotional weight and it doesn't always show up as physical weight. There are people who manage to lose weight without addressing their emotions, but not having worked on their internal issues, they continue their battle with food. There are even some people who never were overweight yet still had a bad association with food and their emotions. For example, I have a friend who has a fantastic, trim figure. But if a boyfriend breaks up with her, she goes off and eats three trays of tempura sushi, locks herself in the house without going to the gym, pounds one sleeve of cookies after another, all to fill the void her broken relationship left behind. It may not affect her weight, but it's clear she has a problem with emotional eating.

Her emotions are completely tied to food. If she doesn't take the time to heal her soul, she will always turn to food in times of struggle.

> *If you run to the pantry every time you have a problem . . . your thoughts, emotions, and feelings are overweight.*

If you run to the pantry every time you have a problem—when you're alone, when you've had a bad day at school, when you have a fight with your boyfriend or your children—your thoughts, emotions, and feelings are overweight. You will only start healing when you stop attacking your body and set aside that irrational guilt. A person with healthy emotions, who doesn't suffer from emotional weight, is a person who feels free and understands that food and emotions shouldn't be tied together. And they show it every day.

The truth is a lot of us have this chubby little voice inside our heads that talks to us and leads us to decisions that increase our emotional weight—and this usually leads to physical weight gain. It's that little voice that tempts you to eat another slice of cake you don't need, that makes you react defensively even when no one is attacking you, that tells you you're worthless when you feel rejected. In the course of reading this book, you'll learn where that little voice comes from, how to make peace with it, understand it, and even love it.

Your best friends in this journey toward health are the 7 steps we'll explore in the next part of the book. These steps will help you reduce the emotional weight that torments you today and, over time, can also help you in other aspects of your life. The result is the healthy body you've always desired. These are the 7 steps we must take to make any major changes in our lives. They are:

1. Make a commitment to yourself
2. Identify your emotional weight
3. Set your goals
4. Affirm your well-being
5. Visualize your desires
6. Take action and create lasting habits
7. Focus on the present

"How can something so simple be so difficult?" you might ask. It's only difficult because we are not regularly aware of these steps. We don't keep them in the forefront of our mind in our day-to-day lives because we don't make a commitment to ourselves. We don't want to acknowledge the problem that is affecting our life, and that prevents us from having enough hope to make goals, affirmations, and visualizations. But once you understand these steps and make them a part of your daily life, and use them not just in times of happiness but in difficult moments, your perspective will completely change. What you once thought impossible will be achievable.

> *All you need is patience, perseverance,*
> *and, of course, ACTION.*

All you need is patience, perseverance, and, of course, ACTION. There may be times when you are tempted to give up, when the climb ahead seems too steep. There will be times when you think you will never manage this change. But I am here to tell you that you can. I am here to encourage you, support you, and tell you to keep fighting because I *know* it's possible. You are not alone. I'm right here beside you, supporting you all the way. I went through all those feelings and challenges. I climbed that mountain myself, through trial and error. I fell many times, but the most important thing is to get back up and keep going. I didn't quit until I discovered these 7 steps, which finally helped me succeed.

These 7 steps are what helped me become the person I am today. That's why I have so much faith that if you allow yourself, if you follow the formula to the T, they will also help you. The power to change your life, to reduce your emotional weight, to heal your soul, is within you and only you. No one can make you go on a diet, follow a plan, and break your own vicious cycle if you are not willing to do it. To achieve this, to finally make this necessary change in your life, you have to take the first step on your own. The fact that you are reading these pages is a sign that you're on the right track: You have to make a commitment to yourself.

(FOUR)

Step 1: Make a Commitment to Yourself

I'M GOING TO lose weight for my daughter's wedding. I'm going to lose weight so I can fit into my dress. I'm going to lose weight for my own wedding. I'm going to lose weight because the man I'm in love with told me to. I'm going to lose weight because I want to be accepted and I want my friends to like me. I'm going to lose weight to appease my parents. Those of us who are overweight have all said things like this to ourselves at some point in our lives. Can you see what each one has in common? None of them is asking you to *commit to yourself*. All these reasons come from the outside. And over the long term, they don't work as effective inspiration: the party is over after a day, the dress goes out of style, boyfriends come and go. All of these reasons are fleeting. But the pain in your heart isn't.

Believe me, doing this because of someone else won't be enough. That type of commitment is too easy to break because you're the only one who is going to be faced with not having that donut or skipping that drink or going to the gym. Setting a goal for yourself is the only way you'll succeed.

This commitment is invisible, yet you can feel it when it's there. You instantly know who is in and who is out. It's time to be honest with yourself, to try to understand what is holding you back and break through to take that important first step. Because, you know what? If you don't do it, no one else will do it for you. The same way you can't make a commitment for someone else, no one else can make this commitment except you. It's that simple. The power is in your hands.

According to a University of Scranton study, 75 percent of those who make a New Year's resolution manage to keep it at least for a week. After four weeks, that number drops to 64 percent. By six months, it's down to 46 percent. After one year, only 39 percent of those twenty-one and over have stuck with their resolution. For those over fifty, it's only 14 percent. Most people never stick with their New Year's resolutions because they don't make a commitment to themselves. They are mere illusions. Commit to yourself and begin to discover who you really are.

Perfect example: I have a friend who wants to write a book. She's in the perfect position to make it happen and has all the tools she needs within her reach. I got together with her. We talked about the subject, developed some ideas, she met with her therapist, her spiritual advisor, her numerologist . . . She did everything in her power to make sure she was on the right path and they all told her to go for it. One of them even gave her a plan of attack: Dedicate half an hour every day to writing until you reach the finish line. She was totally equipped to begin. She'd made all her assurances. All she had to do was finally take action. I was super excited for her. I wanted to encourage her and I wanted to know how it was going. So a couple of weeks later I called her and asked.

"So, how's the book going?"

"I started right in on the first day," she said. "And then I set it aside. It's just that I'm so busy! I had to take my daughter to soccer practice and my son needed me to buy him some notebooks for school. Then my husband asked me to a work event, and my parents came into town to visit. I've been so busy . . ."

I stopped paying attention. Excuses, excuses, and more excuses. I realized she'd taken all the necessary steps except the crucial first one: to commit to herself. That's why this is the first of the 7 steps. If you don't make a commitment to yourself, you'll never achieve everything that's within your reach.

I know another woman who is very overweight. She's always tired, sweating, and she's constantly struggling to breathe. She even breathes heavily through her mouth to take in more oxygen. I know exactly what she's feeling on the inside and outside. Not only does she have to carry around all that excess physical weight, she has to carry around the emotional weight inside. The outside reflects the inside. She's a wonderful person and she knows she's overweight, so much so that she's even told me she doesn't think she has much longer to live, because some days she can barely get out of bed. And she laughs—to cover up her pain, she treats it as a joke.

Regardless, however hard it is for her to get out of a chair, when there's food involved, she's the first one at the table, serving herself a huge plate to ease her pain. I see her and I see myself years ago. I understand her. But I also know there's absolutely nothing I can do to help her if she doesn't commit to helping herself. Happiness and the ability to lose that excess weight are in her hands and her hands only. But as long as she treats it as one big joke, as long as she hides behind laughter and excuses, she'll never reach her goal.

ENOUGH EXCUSES!

I want you to stop for a moment right now and be totally honest with yourself: When you fail to meet a goal, do you justify it with excuses? Do you use your kids, job, spouse, parents, brothers and sisters, friends, uncles, or school as the reason you haven't made the change you desire?

I don't care about all the reasons why you didn't do what you said you wanted to. It doesn't affect my life in the least that you haven't made that change or that you haven't confronted your emotional weight. The only person it truly affects is you, and you alone. You're the only one impacted by this physical and emotional weight. Don't you think you deserve to make yourself a priority? Don't you deserve to be happy? Aren't you allowed to fulfill your dreams? If you answered "no" to any of those three questions, I want you to change your answer right now to a resounding "YES!" Yes, you do deserve to make yourself a priority. Yes, you deserve to be happy. Yes, you deserve to reach your dreams. It all starts with this first step.

> *You're the only one impacted by this physical and emotional weight.*

Once you commit to yourself, you set aside all your excuses. You give yourself the importance that you deserve, and you go from victim to hero in your own life. Justifying the reason you haven't taken that first step doesn't help in the least. It's time you take the bull by the horns and take back control of your life. You can't spend your life blaming others when the ability to change things is in your hands. The moment you commit to yourself, you're immediately in control of whatever has been keeping you down. That's why this is the first step on your path to healing.

> *The commitment to yourself is the first step toward freedom and finding the space you need to finally focus on your dreams.*

The commitment to yourself is the first step toward freedom and finding the space you need to finally focus on your dreams. Because emotional weight is a distraction so great that it does not allow you to focus on anything else, it doesn't allow you to live the life that you deserve. All your energy becomes focused on that excess baggage, on that suffering, on the conflict you have been carrying around for so long. Until you make the decision to help yourself, you won't get very far.

PLACE YOUR NAME AMONG YOUR PRIORITIES

The key toward taking each of the 7 steps we're discussing in this book lies within you. Identifying your emotional weight, finding your willpower, setting goals, creating affirmations, visualizing your good health, taking action, and focusing on the present are all within your reach. But in order to do so, you need to discover that internal strength, the one stronger than all the false beliefs you've been dragging around since childhood. Remember: The universe favors the brave.

Remember: The universe favors the brave.

But that's also the reason why this can be a very difficult step. Those beliefs ingrained in our heads since childhood are hard to shake. As children, we learn to put others' needs before our own. Your mother guilted you into eating your whole plate because she'd spent two hours cooking it or she'd invoke the starving children of Africa who would give anything to have your plate of food. Your father told you to study because he'd sacrificed such long hours at work to pay for your school. Your teacher, your aunt, your grandmother—people throughout your life have said things like this to you and you felt guilty if you didn't obey. Especially in the Latino culture I grew up in, we were taught to serve others, respect our elders, and never say no. We teach women to be homemakers who should dedicate their entire lives to their children and their husbands. We're so accustomed to sacrificing our needs and wants for others' sake that doing something for ourselves can be new and even terrifying. What's more, sometimes we even hide behind this fear of the unknown, clinging to our problems and drifting further from our desires because we are afraid of our own power or success.

For example, a woman who has been the victim of sexual abuse might gain weight subconsciously so that men won't be attracted to her, to hide her sexuality, to repel the opposite sex. Then, when her mother might say, "Baby, why haven't you gotten married yet?" the daughter can answer, "Because I'm fat." End of story. She places the blame on her weight. She uses the excuse to get her mom out of her hair. But inside, she suffers in silence. The memory of that pain lives on in her mind. Her weight gain becomes a further punishment. No one—not her mother, not her best friend, no one—can heal her heart for her.

> *A commitment that stems from an obligation to another person is not a lasting one.*

A commitment that stems from an obligation to another person is not a lasting one. Not only do you have to do it for yourself, you have to give it everything you've got. Any time you undertake a new project—be it a new business, going to school, a new relationship, moving to a new city—you have to put all your heart, all your will, all your time and energy toward it. That's how you achieve extraordinary results. The secret is in being able to exercise self-control, in focusing on the task at hand and giving it all your discipline.

To strengthen your will, you have to train your brain into realizing that a winner's greatest attribute is an abundance of discipline. Willpower is what makes you follow through on your word to keep that commitment to yourself. It's the greatest virtue of passionate, successful people. When I see a person who is overweight, I know what that person is going through, because I lived it. I know very well the control that excess weight exercises over a person's life. But I also know that every person has the willpower to keep it from controlling his or her own life. Yes, that includes you. You can turn the page and take back your power. You *can* stop punishing yourself. You *can* remove that excess weight one piece of baggage at a time and heal your heart and mind. The excess weight—both on the inside and out—is just another form of mistreating yourself. That feeling that you're worthless leads you to eat more and more. You see it as the ideal refuge, that food is the only thing that understands you and can bring you happiness. But all you're doing is abusing your body, mind, and spirit.

When you reach this point, those French fries, cakes, and cookies are like a shot of heroin feeding your addiction. I understand you. You become so used to that pain that you see no way out. You feel this dark room you're living in will be like this forever. I know, because it happened to me. I was so desperate that I started contemplating suicide. Meanwhile, my rage was like a volcano, waiting to erupt when I least expected it. It wasn't until I weighed 314 pounds that I found the strength to finally make a commitment to myself.

WILLPOWER IS YOUR BEST FRIEND

Willpower is one of nature's greatest virtues. And the good news is that if you feel like you've lacked willpower until now, you can learn to develop it. It will give you a great sense of freedom and independence since you'll stop being a slave to your impulses, your past, and your old, painful beliefs.

To make a commitment to yourself, you have to reach the point where the pain of your situation propels you to find a cure. It's like waking up with a mild headache. At first, you may not pay much attention to it, hoping it will go away. But if it gets worse after a couple of hours, you might take Advil until you can see the doctor. These moments, when we reach a point where we can't take it anymore, are the ones that lead us to find a cure. They make us look for a solution, once and for all. It's what leads us to finally make that commitment to ourselves.

The desire to feel better is what leads us down the path to success in all areas of our lives. That's what will eventually put you in the right place. It's what will help you take the next step to continue curing your emotional health. And you will achieve it with your own willpower, with your desire to change, to feel better, to heal yourself. Without that willpower, most likely you won't get very far. That's why when people ask me to help their son or daughter lose weight, I respond, "Until he or she is ready to make that change, it's never going to happen."

What is willpower? You can't buy it in a pill or a bottle. Willpower is that desire inside that drives our ambition. It's truly an extraordinary force that can help us overcome obstacles. It's that inner drive that carries us forward to face and overcome any barrier in the way of us and our goals. The good news is that we can develop and strengthen our willpower if we understand where it comes from and why we haven't done a better job of helping it blossom.

Having willpower means delaying gratification and resisting temptation in the short term so we might achieve results over the long term. Willpower means being able to control your impulses and emotions without being ruled by them. It's self-control over the mind, body, and spirit. At first, doing something you don't like might seem hard, but actually *doing* it despite fear and frustration is the perfect training to develop willpower. The more you exercise discipline, the more accustomed you'll be to taking the right path.

The more you exercise discipline,
the more accustomed you'll be
to taking the right path.

Taking action helps us break down bad habits that have derailed our goals in the past, be it weight loss or any other objective. Willpower doesn't have a mind of its own. It only awaits your instructions. Learn to control it so you can achieve that strength. Decide to do the things you *have* to do. Simply start and you'll see what you're able to accomplish in a matter of weeks. Every time you face your fears bravely and take action, your willpower grows. Small victories become large ones. That's the key to maintaining that commitment to yourself. You need something to get you into action. It's a force much greater than the excess weight that's holding you back. Connect with your inner willpower; it's inside you! Toss aside your excuses and make the commitment today!

THE DEEP PAIN THAT SPURRED MY CHANGE

Between my 314 pounds, the constant ridicule at school and around town, and the dark thoughts I was having about suicide, I told myself, "If I'm really that fat, if I'm really so worthless, then I ought to do what people say: diet." And that's how I began my foray into the world of dieting. Although I hadn't yet made that commitment to myself, I was getting closer to taking that fundamental first step. I knew I was too heavy. And I knew that if I did nothing about it, one day I'd be unable even to get out of bed.

Since dieting for a man was considered taboo in my country back in the '90s, I started it in secret, hidden from my parents. In a Hispanic-Arabic family, being a big, strong, stocky man was synonymous with masculinity. I started looking for answers in my mother's celebrity gossip magazines, where all the men and women had phenomenal bodies and seemed to have perfect lives. The interviewers would ask the celebrities what they did to remain so trim, and all of them said that it was genetics, that they eat whatever they wanted and barely exercised. I was confused. I couldn't understand how a person could look that good while eating whatever they wanted, while I was the exact opposite. I asked God why He had punished me like this. I didn't realize it then, but I was getting ready to take the first step, albeit not using the healthiest or most advisable method.

One time I read that to lose weight, some Asians used mesotherapy, which consists of treating the affected fat areas with microinjections, homeopathic medicines, vitamins, etc. It seemed like an easy method and like something I could do in secret in my room without anyone being the wiser. Bingo! I went running to my neighborhood Eastern medicine store to buy everything I needed for the treatment. I locked myself in my room and got to work—without any help or guidance. It was so dangerous that to this day I still have a mark where I contracted an infection at the injection site. I hurt myself and it didn't help me lose weight. But my emotional pain and suffering from my weight was so great that nothing deterred me.

Another time, I heard about a special girdle and special cream that could help anyone lose weight. Another magical solution: let's give it a shot! Every morning, I'd wake up, spread that special warming cream all over my belly, and strap on the girdle as tight as possible. It was supposed to melt away the fat. Then, I put on my regular school clothes and, of course, the damn sweater, which was my armor against the rest of the world. I sweat a lot to begin with, but now, with the cream and the girdle, it was unbearable. It was uncomfortable, my skin was on fire, all for the sake of losing weight. After a few days of this, in Maturín's simmering weather, I soon developed a terrible rash all over my stomach. Another wasted effort.

Meanwhile, my weight had reached the point where everything was a struggle: Getting out of bed, putting on my underwear, my shoes, my T-shirt. Falling asleep took forever. The simple act of lying down in bed became a struggle as I tossed and turned to find a comfortable position where I could breathe well. Only then could I fall asleep. Even showering was a challenge. How do you dry yourself, your feet, if you can't reach them? When I finally managed to dry off one side of my body, the other side was already sweaty from the effort. I considered taking another shower. But what for? To repeat the same process all over again? I spent my life feeling hot. All I wanted was to be in an air-conditioned room. And my God, the smell! I felt like I smelled horrible, like fat and sweat. It got to the point where I showered three times a day. And no matter how much cologne I put on, the smell was always there.

When I was a young boy, before I was overweight, my mother—like all mothers—would ask me if I'd already taken a shower and brushed my teeth. I would absentmindedly say, "Yeah, yeah," as I continued playing Nintendo, and she believed me, even if I hadn't showered. But once, years later when I was grossly overweight, my mother asked me the same question. But this time, though I had actually just showered, she replied, "You're lying to me! That's it, I'm going to get my flip flops to teach you a lesson!" She came back into the room with her *chancleta*, and chased me into the bathroom, yelling, stripped off my clothes and put me in the shower. I wanted to die from embarrassment. Beyond the shame of her not believing me, I had hit puberty and was starting to grow hair in all the usual places. Now imagine how mortified I was as she started scrubbing me furiously.

Of course, now I understand what happened. Since I was so big, there were parts of my body I couldn't reach when I showered, like the back of my neck. When my mother saw the filth in the rolls behind my neck, she thought I was lying to her because it looked like I hadn't showered at all. What a terrible and embarrassing moment. I'll never forget it.

All the while, I continued trying to diet in secret. If I heard that bread was fattening, then I'd stop eating bread—but I kept pounding pastries and sodas and rice. Later, I heard that rice was fattening, so I'd tell my mother:

"Mom, I'm not really hungry for rice today," I'd say.

"What? You *have* to eat rice," she'd insist.

"No, no, really. I don't want any."

So instead, she'd serve me a small mountain of potatoes. Obviously, I wasn't going to lose weight eating this way, but I didn't know it at the time. And of course, she didn't know I was trying to lose weight. I treated it like a state secret.

Meanwhile, the bullying and taunting had reached a fever pitch. By my junior year in high school, I didn't even feel like going to school or to the social club. One day, my dad came over to me and asked me what was going on. Finally, I confided in him that I was being mocked and I couldn't take it anymore. He wanted to know if anyone in particular was harassing me, and I told him yes.

The taunting started the second I walked into class. I liked to sit at the front, since learning was important to me. But the abuse was so much that I had to change where I sat. When I sat up front, my classmates would yell out things like, "What does it say on the board, Miss? I can't see with this elephant sitting in front of me!" I started coming in a few minutes late to class and sat in the very last row in the back. I didn't even care if my teachers reprimanded me for being late. I just didn't want to hear it from the other students. How I dreamed I could just become invisible. The biggest problem with my new strategy was that the boy who made the most fun of me, who started right in on me the second I walked into class, also sat in the back row. All I could do was take it and pray for a quick end to the school day.

My father was shocked, because until now, he had no idea I'd been suffering this kind of abuse at school. He told me a story from when he was a boy. There was a kid who sold newspapers on his block and whose sole purpose in life, it seemed, was to make fun of my dad, until one day my father lost it. He grabbed a bottle and shattered it over the kid's head. After that day, the kid never bothered my dad again. He told me there were times in life where you had to fight back to teach the other person a lesson. I listened to him carefully. Never could I have imagined that my dad, my mentor, had suffered similar abuse. Nevertheless, I'd never been physically aggressive toward anyone. I didn't even know how to throw a punch. But my dad's story emboldened me.

This definitely wasn't the right answer to my situation, but I'm sure my father didn't know how else to help me face this fear. He told me this personal story to give me enough courage to go back to school and defend myself. He couldn't have imagined what would happen just a few days later.

After this talk with my dad, he dropped me off at school as usual. I went back to my strategy of going in late. I sat in the last row, at the back of the class, and, sure enough, my bully said to me, "Come on, cow, moo for me. Come on. Do it." I was blinded with years of pent-up rage. Before I realized it, I'd grabbed my pencil, turned around, and stabbed it into his neck. He screamed in pain. Blood spurted from the wound, and the teacher came running to see what had happened. I was frozen, in a trance, snorting like a bull. I'd reached my limit. All I could think was that if anyone else made fun of me, I'd stab them with a pencil, too. I was completely out of my mind. The rage had been building, bubbling under the surface like a volcano, until it erupted and shot molten lava in all directions, regardless of who it injured. All reasoning, sanity, and empathy left me. I reacted with a violence that was completely out of character for me.

They called the ambulance and my father, and they suspended me from school for three days. Thank God, nothing serious happened to the other boy. But it served as a huge wake-up call to my parents. They finally opened their eyes and started to see that there was a serious problem. At the beginning they hadn't seen my weight gain as an issue in and of itself, but they had noticed my aggression. Until that point, I had managed to hurt others with my words but never physically. That's why this episode shocked them. It was time to do something.

They figured that if I managed to lose weight, the taunts at school would stop and I wouldn't be so aggressive anymore. So they bought a book called *The Anti-Diet* and started taking steps to helping me lose weight. The problem with this strategy was that I hadn't yet made a commitment to myself. They were trying to get me to commit by imposing new rules for my well-being, but it all hadn't clicked for me at that point. And until one commits to one's self, everyone else's efforts are in vain. My mother put a lock on the refrigerator and tied a knot only she knew how to loosen around the pantry to try to control my eating. But since I hadn't committed to myself, that lock and knot made no difference to me. I'd go to my dad's work and ask the girl at the cash register for money. She'd write out an IOU, give me the money, and I'd use it to buy whatever I wanted to eat without my parents knowing.

At home, since my parents were conscious of trying to help me lose weight, at least they started paying attention to nutrition and how to incorporate more healthy meals into our daily life. My mother switched out regular mayo for light. Instead of an *arepa*, a hotdog, or a sandwich at night, we ate cornflakes with yogurt and fruit. We ate fruit instead of desserts. And instead of soda, my mother made "natural" juices (with plenty of sugar). But since my sisters were so skinny, my mother ended up having to cook two separate meals, one for them and one for me. My mom and dad started doing the diet along with me to help support me. That change helped me not to feel so alone.

My parents always went on an hour-long walk every morning. To help me, they added an evening walk so that I could go along with them. The major problem is that none of us knew anything about nutrition. They didn't realize how much sugar there was in cereal, yogurt, and fruit. And we didn't know how important portion control was to losing weight. The result was that despite all these changes, I saw no difference whatsoever in my body.

I became obsessed with the scale. Just after our evening

walk, I'd hurry to my parents' room, step on the scale to see how much weight I'd lost, and was disappointed to watch the needle land in the same place. I became consumed with my weight, with my pants size, but I still hadn't made a commitment to myself. My routine became to weigh myself before school while my parents made breakfast, not eat the entire day at school (thinking this would help me lose weight), and then I'd weigh myself again once I got home. Then I'd eat lunch because I was starving, and step on the scale again, relieved to see I hadn't gained weight after eating. Then, I'd diet for three straight days, gain weight, and didn't understand why. The situation was becoming dire. Since I didn't have the correct information, of course I wasn't going to lose any weight. And because I was not losing weight, I'd get discouraged and wonder: *What's the point?*

My parents tried to keep my spirits up so I wouldn't lose hope. Even though I'd never really liked soccer, my father tried to sign me up for a league at the Arab club. He bought me the jersey, shorts, cleats, socks, everything to get me excited about playing. But at 300 pounds, I looked like a joke out there. I showed up to the match disguised as a soccer player and spent the entire time on the bench. I was ashamed to get up and walk off the field after the match. The others were sweaty, dirty, joking among themselves while my uniform was immaculate. Yet another disappointment.

Then my parents tried eliminating all sweets from our house. It started because my grandmother had just been diagnosed with diabetes. My dad got scared and got rid of every last bit of chocolate and dessert so the same thing wouldn't happen to us. But since that was his decision, and I hadn't committed myself to losing weight, I found ways to keep eating sweets. I emptied out a shampoo bottle, filled it with M&Ms, and kept it in my P.E. locker. Even though my dad swore I wasn't having any sweets, each time I had to go to that damn P.E. class, I could at least eat my chocolate in peace. I looked for comfort in chocolate.

Meanwhile, I was getting frustrated. I hated that my legs felt so heavy, that I always felt like my body was in an oven, and that I was constantly sweating. I hated everything I had to do to keep my oversized body functioning. That included having to smear on a special cream where my body parts rubbed together and chafed. Everything was a hassle. Getting dressed. Putting on my shoes. Taking a shower. Wiping myself. Cutting my toenails. It was getting impossible to live with myself.

And that's how I found myself coming to terms on October 27, 1997. That day, the day of my fifteenth birthday, I woke up exhausted from not being able to sleep restfully. I was tired of sweating every day like I was at the beach instead of inside an air-conditioned room. Tired of the taunts. So tired of being tired. And that's when it clicked. I stood in front of the mirror in my underwear and really looked at the body that was causing me so much pain. I became enraged at the reflection I barely recognized, this person who had taken over my body and ruined my life. I looked and felt so heavy I didn't know how I could go on this way. The rage coalesced into a kind of vengeance that stirred from deep down. Suddenly, I thought, *I need to kill this person, I need to murder him. He has to die.* I'd reached my limit. I couldn't take it anymore. I looked directly into my eyes in the mirror and said out loud, "This is where the overweight Alejandro dies."

That's the moment I finally committed to myself. The anger, the exhaustion, the desire to change took over and forced me to take that all-important first step. From that moment on, I was so committed that I no longer regretted turning down a piece of bread. My determination was greater than any piece of cake or chocolate. My anger was stronger than any temptation anyone might put before me. My willpower had finally risen from beyond my folds of fat and the deep sadness that had held me back for so many years. The only thing I wanted, with all my heart and soul, was to get rid of the weight.

THE ROAD TO COMMITMENT

Whenever I go out to eat with a group—since they know my story, my struggle, and the effort it took me to lose weight—they're often embarrassed to admit they'd like to order something off the dessert menu. "Come on, guys. Order all the dessert you want!" I tell them. They become overly conscious of what they're eating because I'm there. Some of them even say, "Sorry, Alejandro, sorry," whenever they eat something fattening. As if I were the patron saint of healthy eating! Everyone is allowed to make his or her own decisions; they don't need to ask me for permission or apologize. Why? Because the most important commitment you can make is not to someone else, but to yourself.

The road to commitment is very personal. Each of us embarks upon the journey in his or her own way. No one can force it upon you. It's something you and only you can do. For example, I can argue with my parents for them to eat more healthfully, but I can't force them to send back the breadbasket at the restaurant. That decision has to come from them. I can't impose my will on them. Because the day they go out to dinner without me, the day I'm not at their side to tell them how to eat healthfully, that's when they have to make their own choices. And if they aren't committed to themselves, they won't make the healthiest decisions. Moreover, if I'm scolding them every time we go out to eat together, they're simply not going to want to go out with me anymore. Each one of us has to make our own commitment to reaching our goals. No one else can do it for us.

Each one of us has to make our own commitment to reaching our goals. No one else can do it for us.

I've made a commitment to myself to eat healthfully and keep my body in shape. I've taken it on and I know what to do to maintain my ideal weight. Some days are easier than others. The other night, for example, I went out to a Spanish restaurant, where they serve delicious chorizo and potatoes and all sorts of delicacies to make your mouth water. I wanted to order the entire menu. But first I asked myself: "Are you willing to pay the price for eating all this or would you rather have the fish and vegetables?" While others pored over the menu, wondering what they were going to order, I continued the conversation with my inner chubby self. "Because if you want to eat all that other stuff, do it, but don't come to me afterward complaining that you shouldn't have and all that other drama." I turned and saw the roasted potatoes arrive at the table next to me. "Go on! You deserve it. Why else do you wake up so early and work so hard? What if you die tomorrow and you didn't get to taste that deliciousness? Why do you deny yourself?" I stayed quiet, still struggling with my inner chubby self, until I won the battle and ordered the fish. It was a personal battle, one only I could fight. How did I win it? Because of my willpower and the commitment I'd made to myself. It's a daily commitment, a decision you make every day when you wake up.

Maybe you think this commitment you're making to yourself today is fleeting, but it isn't. It's for life. I'm healthy, at my ideal weight, but for me, it's one meal at a time. There's always an internal struggle. I talk to the chubby little voice inside my head every time I sit down at a restaurant. It's all about making decisions and having the willpower to keep going down the right path.

Let's be honest, none of us fantasize about eating steamed broccoli with lemon, garlic, olive oil, and parsley. We're programmed to think that for something to be good, it has to be fattening. I think even I, as someone who is accustomed to healthy eating, could never speak passionately about a salad.

We're accustomed to dreaming about food bathed in creamy sauces or sweet, delicious desserts. I'm tempted daily to eat something I shouldn't. But my commitment to myself and my willpower help me make the decisions that make me feel good in the long term.

Now, this doesn't mean I don't have an occasional cheat day. It's possible to break that commitment every now and then, but you have to be aware of it and be ready to get back on track as soon as possible. It's like when you start a diet on a Monday, and by Wednesday, you might find yourself saying, "Oh, one little spoonful of Nutella won't hurt anyone." The next day, you say the same thing—except this time, you eat two spoonfuls. Once you break this commitment with yourself, it's easy to continue breaking it. Remember, habits come from consistent repetition. When you find that it happens to you—because you're human and it happens to all of us—I want you to stop for a moment and really think about what you're doing. Think about the consequences of each of those spoonfuls. Think about all the effort you've been making to keep the commitment to yourself and make a change. Think about how it will affect your life. That will help you refocus on your commitment toward personal healing.

I know that making that commitment to yourself and connecting with your personal pain isn't easy. Maybe you find yourself thinking, *There's no way I can do this. For what? To suffer more than I'm already suffering?* But I'm asking you to do it because it is going to make you feel better than you ever thought possible. Just because you've never made that commitment to yourself, or because you've tried and failed, doesn't mean you can't do it. It's never too late. It doesn't matter what stage you're at in your life. If you really want it, that commitment is within your reach. It's the first of the 7 steps that will take you toward real, lasting change, to reaching your goals, realizing your dreams, and finally embracing happiness.

Essential tips to transform your life

- Include yourself in your list of priorities. If you don't take care of yourself, no one else will.
- Find your inner strength to achieve the change you're seeking for your life.
- Commit to yourself. It's never too late. *Yes, you can!*

Put It into Practice!

A CONTRACT WITH YOURSELF

The commitment is *Yours alone*. It doesn't matter that it's invisible. Your mind knows it and processes it, but making it tangible and seeing it makes it much more powerful. I want you to make this commitment to yourself today, with all the respect and seriousness that you deserve. I want you to be responsible for your own decisions and actions. I want you to decide, once and for all, to take the path toward the happiness that you so deserve. Are you ready to take on this commitment and reach your goals? If your answer is "yes," sign the contract with yourself below and date it.

Today, I make a commitment to myself to heal myself, inside and out, to unload the excess baggage in my life and cure my emotional weight, to live the happy and healthy life that I deserve.

______________________________ _______________

SIGNATURE DATE

Now that you've signed your contract, I want you to read it again and really look at it. Look at your signature and recognize what the words mean. Close your eyes, think about your goal, put your hand over your heart, and feel the passion in it right now. That's your power, your strength, your willpower. Smile and promise to do everything necessary to change your life. Everything is in your hands now. Everything depends on you and no one else. You can no longer blame your circumstances, your past, or your parents. There are no more excuses. Every time you are tempted to break your commitment, because it happens to all of us, think back to this contract and your signature on this page. Reread it, reconnect with the power of your word, remember how important you are, and continue on the path toward happiness.

Betty Escalona

I'm Betty Escalona. I'm Venezuelan and I'm thirty years old. Life dealt me a terrible surprise when my first daughter, Victoria, was born with spina bifida. A year and a half later my daughter Valeria was born, and, together, they are a blessing in my life. It hasn't been easy. As a single mother, I left my home country to come to Houston so that my angel could receive the treatments she requires. I tried to drown all my sadness, fears, and lack of love in food until I weighed 183 pounds.

When Victoria stopped breathing one day, watching her fight for her life, I realized I couldn't keep on being overweight, exhausted, and bitter. I needed to be healthy to be there for my loved ones.

Watching Despierta América, *I was inspired by my fellow Venezuelan Alejandro Chabán, and thanks to Yes You Can! I've lost forty-five pounds, going from a size 14 to a size 6 with a completely healthy plan. This victory is both for and because of my daughter!*

SUCCESS STORY

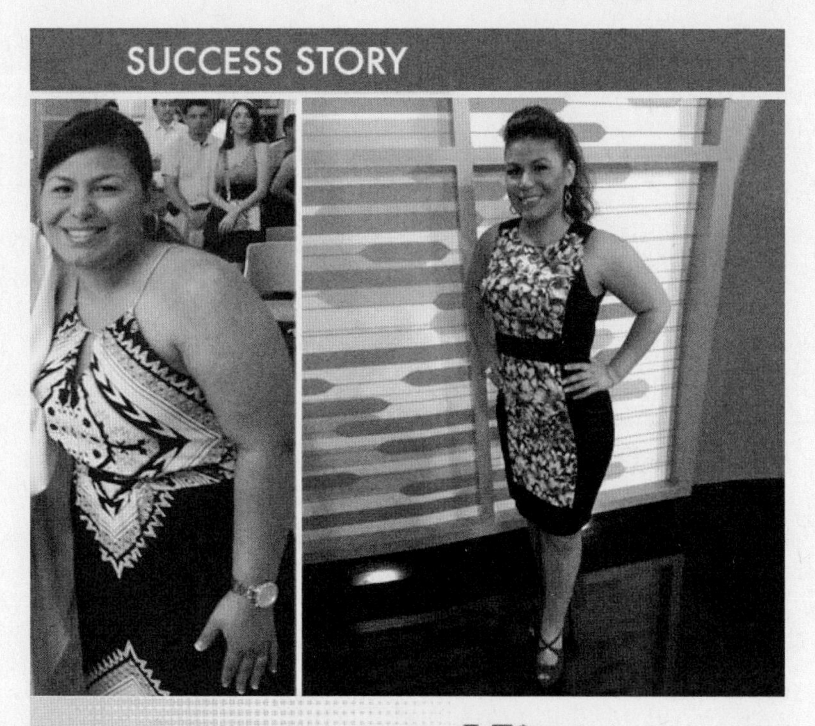

BETTY ESCALONA lost 45* lbs

BETTY'S ADVICE: *What helped me reach my goal was watching how hard my daughter—who is in a wheelchair and nearly died three times when she stopped breathing—fought for her life. My daughter Victoria has won every battle she's faced, and in her, I found my strength.*

**Results not typical and will vary according to diet, exercise, metabolism, and genetic makeup.*

(FIVE)

Step 2: Identify Your Emotional Weight

WHAT DOES IT mean to identify your emotional weight? How do we take this important step? Where to start? I think the first thing you have to do is reconnect with your emotions and your reactions to different situations to see what makes you eat when you're not actually hungry. Now, I know this can be an uncomfortable step. I can understand why you don't want to open up this trunk where you're storing all that baggage filled with your toxic and painful emotions. But it's important to understand what you're dealing with so that you can take another step toward healing your soul and finding the freedom and happiness you deserve.

> *It's important to understand what you're dealing with so that you can take another step toward healing your soul.*

Do you know why it's so important to identify your emotional weight? Because it will open up the path so that you can finally find the internal peace you need to reach your goals and your biggest dreams. If you don't identify the root of your problem you'll never be able to grow strong, healthy habits. For example, a friend decided to make a commitment to herself and do whatever was necessary to lose the hundred pounds that had been weighing her down for years. She signed up to Yes You Can! and in the course of a year and a half, she lost seventy pounds. She felt and looked like a goddess. She had committed to herself and achieved her goal. However, in the process, she didn't pay attention to her emotional weight. She skipped that step in the plan and went right to the nutrition, movement, and supplements. She didn't stop to identify and discover the origins of her problem so that she could begin healing her soul.

What was affecting her? Her entire life, she'd been her mommy's little girl. Her mom would defend her weight gain, she would cook for her so she wouldn't feel so bad about her obesity, she would drive her to and from places, and it went on like this until she turned forty. Tired of being single and wanting to get married and have children, she started losing weight. Once she was thinner, she started to feel confident for the first time and started going out on dates—she was one step closer to realizing her desires. Everything was going fine until her mother started manipulating her with words: "You never spend time with us anymore. Your grandmother doesn't see you on the weekends. I'm up all night waiting for you to come home. What if something bad happens to us? You're out all night with a different guy and you don't care about your family anymore." Little by little, those words started eating away at her, making her feel guilty. She'd always given everything for her family. She'd dedicated her life to her mother and her grandmother, and they'd created a codependent relationship. But when she took flight and started building her own life, her mother felt that her daughter was abandoning her and she began to manipulate her.

Since my friend hadn't managed to resolve the emotional issues that led her to gain weight, she fell into the trap, started to feel like a victim, the guilty party, and started thinking herself a bad daughter. Do you know what was happening to her? She was scared to be happy—scared to finally reach her goal and start living the unknown, a life on her own. Her guilt returned and with it came the pounds. Her wounded heart started to hurt once again. Little by little, she began gaining back all the weight that she'd fought so hard to lose. Not only had she broken the commitment to herself, she had never identified her emotional weight. She didn't stop to work on her emotions, didn't discover the root of her problem, didn't reinforce her self-esteem and heal the wounds of the past—and ultimately she ended up back where she started.

The problems start inside us, in our hearts and souls. If we don't uncover the reason behind why we eat badly, no diet will ever work. To change what's on the outside, first we have to change what's on the inside.

> *To change what's on the outside,*
> *first we have to change what's on the inside.*

Identifying your emotional weight—that heaviness that prevents you from growing in the ways you deserve—means taking stock of what you're *feeling*. It means connecting with the chubby self you carry around inside you. It means truly understanding why that chubby self drives you to be self-destructive with your body and your life. The only way to make real change and improve your life is to take stock of what has been hurting you inside, look at it, accept it, and understand it. Listen to yourself. What's more, if you find yourself plateaued on a diet, it's very possible that your emotions are preventing you from breaking through that plateau.

PAY ATTENTION TO YOUR BEHAVIOR

Emotional weight is something so individual, so personal. It has so much to do with our own intimate stories that it's almost impossible to come up with a comprehensive list of all the things that can cause these emotional shortcomings. Nevertheless, eating until we burst, using drugs to lose ourselves, drinking until we're out of control are all extreme forms of addiction that we use to fill a void or cover up some kind of pain. They are methods we use to hide from the reality of our lives. Sometimes, this emotional weight is so deeply rooted inside us that we keep coming back to these harmful behaviors again and again—even while knowing that this pleasure is only a brief respite before more pain, anguish, and regret. Nevertheless, we do it over and over.

The problem is we're tying to find a physical solution to a mental, spiritual, and emotional problem. We go back to that carton of ice cream. If you're upset over a relationship that's ended, over the death of a loved one, the loss of a job, you end up back on the couch with that carton of ice cream and eat the whole thing. Does your sadness magically disappear? No. Actually, what usually happens to all of us is that we're hit with another, stronger wave of sadness because now we don't feel well physically, either. Our stomach hurts because of all the ice cream, we feel heavy, we know it's not good for us, so to the sadness we add guilt and remorse. Not only have we not solved anything, we've added more toxic emotions to the mix.

Not healing your emotional weight is like being in a constant battle with your well-being.

Not healing your emotional weight is like being in a constant battle with your well-being. Here are some other examples:

- It's like if you get fired from your job and then you spend night after night going to the bar to drown your sorrows in alcohol. You won't feel any better the next morning. On the contrary, not only will you still be upset at losing your job, now your head will hurt for having drunk so much, there will be less money in your pocket, and you'll have done nothing to solve your problem—the solution is to look for a new job.

- It's like if your girlfriend breaks up with you and the first thing you do is go down to the corner store, buy yourself a pack of cigarettes, and smoke the entire pack, one by one. When you've finished that last cigarette, not only will you realize your ex-girlfriend still hasn't called, but now your lungs feel heavy, your throat hurts, you smell like an ashtray, and it's harder to breathe. This action didn't improve your situation at all. You're still sad and upset, but now you've put your health at risk, too.
- It's like if you get into an argument with your husband and you rush off to the mall to buy new clothes and purses and shoes to give yourself a moment of joy. But those purchases don't solve the root of your problem. By the time you get home, see everything you've bought and put it all away, you realize that the heaviness in your heart remains. Not only that, now you have more clothes than you know what to do with—and more debt.

The same thing happens when we turn to the food in our refrigerator as a refuge. We eat anything and everything to mask our pain, but that brief moment of pleasure solves nothing and only packs on more pounds. Now we not only have to deal with the pain that led us to eat, but with extra physical weight we now have to lose. And if losing weight is your ultimate goal, then you've done nothing but put an obstacle in your own path. You've made your journey that much harder.

The emotional weight that rules your life is like a speaker playing music. You can put clothes on top of it to drown out the noise, but that won't stop the music. Maybe you can't hear it for a while or at points throughout the day, but when you try to go to sleep, in the stillness of the night, you'll hear music in the distance—a sad and unavoidable melody.

Lying there, with the buzz of the music swirling around your room in the darkness, you have two options. You can turn over, ignore it, and try to keep sleeping or you can get out of bed and do something about it. Identifying your emotional weight is like deciding to get out of bed, taking the clothes off the speaker, and hearing the music in full. You'll recognize the song immediately. Listen to it carefully. Every lyric, every phrase has something to say about your past, maybe a past you've tried to forget. Maybe it will make you sad. But you have to face it, accept it, and recognize it. Only by doing this can you, after hard work, turn this into a more pleasant melody. Because you'll finally have the power to change the station to music that instead of making you feel sad, makes you feel like dancing. But that can only happen if you listen to the melody playing in your soul. You must identify it, accept it, forgive it, love it, and work to change it.

WHAT ARE YOU PROTECTING YOURSELF FROM?

When you swallow your feelings, you're protecting yourself from pain, trauma, or a frustration you're carrying inside your heart and mind. I ate to fill a void but I hadn't realized my emotions played a role in all this. I just thought I was using food to cover my pain.

Even though I was told of all the damage my obesity was doing to me physically, I couldn't picture all the damage it was doing to my mind and body. It wasn't tangible. What was tangible was that slice of cake that soothed my anxiety, the chocolate that alleviated my anguish, the ice cream that froze my desire to break down into tears. Eating protected me from my fears. Recently, during psychotherapy sessions, I started to discover that key connection between how I felt and what I ate. I understood it better as I worked on my emotions in the following years, and as I continue to work on it.

Listen to your body. When your body is pushed to extremes, it asks for help, screams for it. It yells out exactly what is unbalanced in your life. But if you don't stop to listen, the root of the unbalance will never be resolved. First you have to become cognizant of the issue and then act.

Stop for a minute. I want you to give yourself the space to reconnect with your emotions. It's the best way to discover which one of them is out of balance and why.

The next time you have a ravenous craving for a *tres leches* cake, nachos slathered in cheese, or a box of donuts, please stop for a second and ask yourself these questions:

- What am I feeling right now?
- Am I anxious?
- Am I frustrated?
- Am I upset?
- Am I sad?
- Am I scared?
- Am I angry?
- Am I actually hungry or is one of these emotions goading me into eating to calm myself?

I want you to ask yourself these questions so you can begin connecting your emotions with your actions. Once you connect the two, it will be easier to identify your emotional weight and to begin taking the steps to unlatch food from your emotions. That way, you can replace the act of eating with a healthier activity that can help you deal with what you're feeling instead of covering it up.

Once you identify the emotions tied to your eating, you can ask yourself other essential questions:

- Which is the emotion that most prompts me to eat?
- Which is the source of the pain, the toxic emotion, that forces me to act this way?
- Why do I think I have to run to food for reassurance?
- What am I protecting myself from?

It's fundamental for you to identify your trigger, the gun that goes off in your hand when you open that carton of ice cream or when your mouth opens for that spoonful of cheesecake. Taking stock of your reactions, analyzing the "why" and "when" it happens, will help you identify the root of your problem. And that will give you the chance to find the better path toward healing your emotional weight, once and for all.

YOU ARE YOUR OWN WORST ENEMY

Over the years, especially since I started Yes You Can!, I've come to realize that many people live backward. They complain, but they aren't compelled to fix the root of their problem—they aren't even interested in identifying it. Many will start a diet only to complain about the menu. They don't like chicken cooked this way or that way; they don't like vegetables or salad; they hate they can't have their glass of wine every single night; they miss cheese. They come up with every excuse to set their diet aside. The problem is they don't understand that they need to identify why it is they are eating, what forces them to eat this way, and what is keeping them from losing weight.

Another typical scenario is when a person who is fifty pounds overweight has been dieting for only a week and has spent that week cheating with a spoonful here, a couple French fries there—and they know it—but they complain that they're seeing no difference on the scale. Instead of being honest with themselves and admitting they have been cheating on their diet and that's the reason they're not losing weight. Instead of trying to identify why they're overeating, they fall back on the classic excuse: "This diet doesn't work." They go back to eating their old way and never get to the crux of the issue. You can't expect drastic changes overnight when it took years to build up what you're carrying around in your body and your soul. No one gains fifty pounds in a week. So you can't expect to lose it in a week, either. The same goes for emotions. Emotional weight accrues inside us over time, and it takes time to heal an injured heart. You need to be patient with yourself. You have to be nurturing to yourself. You have to learn to like yourself, to love yourself, instead of punishing yourself for every mistake you make. If you slip on your diet, if you veer off course, make a correction and keep moving forward on your journey.

> *You can't expect drastic changes overnight when it took years to build up what you're carrying around in your body and your soul.*

When you finally discover the root of your problem and identify your emotional weight, you'll be able to ease that pain, anxiety, fear, and sadness with new tools. You'll finally be able to change the meaning of those emotions, write a new story for yourself, and feel the peace and joy you deserve.

THE RED ALERT THAT SAVED MY LIFE

I was suffering from my emotions—sadness, anger, fear—in their rawest form when I finally made a commitment to myself to kill off fat Alejandro. But I hadn't yet realized everything

I was feeling was related to my weight. I felt so many things without knowing where they came from. I didn't know how to control my emotions or how they affected me. I didn't have the information I needed to be cognizant of any of this. In my family—and in others of that time—you didn't sit down to analyze your problems. In my Hispanic culture, there's very little information about nutrition and the reason for weight gain. You simply live with it. If we don't understand the "why," we'll never be able to solve the problem.

When I finally committed to myself and decided it was time to get serious about losing weight, I used the method of trial and error. Instead of eating that piece of cake I was craving, I'd run off to the nature store and buy a bag of granola—without understanding that if I ate *the entire bag* it wasn't going to be any better. I ate dried fruits, not knowing that they were loaded with sugar, instead thinking it was healthier than eating a sugary snack. I started going to the gym and even taking all kinds of diet pills with ephedrine, which at the time was sold without fully understanding its dangerous side effects. Those first few days on a diet seemed to last an eternity. I thought that so much effort meant I'd see results fast. But with so much weight to lose and so few days on any one diet—not to mention the fact that I was making up my own diet as I went along—results were slow to come.

It felt like all my effort and sacrifices weren't paying off. So in the following months, I decided to take drastic measures. My mother made my breakfast—usually an *arepa* with ham and cheese—which I would take with me to school and throw away before class. When I got home, I'd eat whatever my mother made for lunch, and the rest of the day, I'd drink nothing but water. I'd go to the gym and when I'd come home, instead of eating dinner, I'd only drink more water. I'd go to bed and the next day, again, I'd have nothing but water until lunch.

By the second or third day that I'd been eating only once a day, I finally started feeling a difference in my body. I don't think it would have been a noticeable change, but I felt lighter. Nevertheless, I'd get dizzy, my head hurt, and I had no energy at all. The fact that I felt lighter meant I kept up this pace for another day, another week, another month, until one day I realized my clothes were getting looser. But I had no idea of the toll it was taking on my health.

With every pound I lost, I gained another pound of emotional weight. I was anxious inside, so much so that I started biting my nails badly. I'd bite my nails to the quick. I even started eating Chapstick—yes, Chapstick! From what I'd heard, it had no calories but it had a syrupy flavor that satisfied my desire for something sweet. At night, if I felt overly weak after eating only one meal in the day, I'd eat a few pieces of papaya. I'd heard that papaya helped you go to the bathroom, so I figured if I was going to eat something, it might as well be something that would help me continue to lose weight. I ate so much papaya that my hands started turning yellowish orange. Neither my parents nor I noticed that my obsession over losing weight was becoming an eating disorder.

Meanwhile, I kept losing weight, and watched as my waist size dropped from 38 to 36 to 34 to 32. Little by little, I started to feel "normal," so to speak. Gosh, I hate that word, because it suggests that people who are overweight are "abnormal," and that's just not the case! At this point, my physical change was noticeable to others. The positive comments never stopped. "You look so thin! Wow, you look great!" Regardless, I wasn't eating right. I looked good on the outside, but my body and soul continued to suffer. Plus no one knew the drastic diet I was on.

It's important to stop here so we can address the fact that I was still missing the key factor to my weight loss: identifying and dealing with my emotional weight. I was eliminating the physical weight, but the emotional weight I'd been carrying around for years was only growing. My body was crying out for help but I ignored it. I looked the other way and focused on my thinner self and the positive comments I was getting, ignoring the fact that something was terribly wrong.

I started getting bruises all over my body. But instead of telling my parents or a doctor, I simply covered them up with clothes—yes, including those blasted sweaters, which I still wore to cover up my insecurities. And even though I had no idea what was going on with me (I even worried it might be skin cancer), I chose to stay quiet, fearing they wouldn't let me keep dieting the way that had helped me lose so much weight. Anything that threatened my newfound slenderness was my mortal enemy; I was terrified of being obese again.

When dinnertime came around, my parents started to say, "Sit down and eat. You haven't eaten a thing all day and your grandmother is worried that you're too skinny. Look at the dark circles under your eyes!" To appease them, I'd sit down to eat, only to end up going to the bathroom later and throwing it all up on purpose. They were right, I'd noticed the dark circles. But I preferred those and the constant weakness over gaining weight again. I started using a concealer for dark circles I found in my sisters' bathroom. If they didn't see the dark circles, they couldn't force me to eat, and that way, everybody won. Or so I thought.

At one point, my body was under so much stress because of my diet that I started to lose my hair. It scared me, but still I kept on with my diet; nothing could replace the sensation of being thinner and seeing that reflected in others' reactions toward me. Jeers became cheers, and all I wanted was to keep losing weight—because I still didn't see myself as thin. Even though I could now wear the "cool" clothes other kids wore, when I looked in the mirror, I still wasn't satisfied. What I saw was someone covered in stretch marks and cellulite, the hanging chest muscles, the saggy skin that hung over my body. It's not what I imagined being thin would be like. All of this saggy, loose skin frustrated me and made me think I had to keep losing although I'd already reached my ideal weight.

Meanwhile, although I lived in a hot climate, I was always cold and slept too much because I was tired all the time. Of course, I had no idea this was because I wasn't consuming enough calories. And since I was near the end of high school, my parents rarely went into my room to see any hints of my sickness. I was still upset at the world; as a result, I was talking back and slamming doors, so much so that my parents tried to respect my space to see if that made any difference. But that only meant they were further estranged from my reality. They had no idea I still wore sweaters to cover up my bruising, that I told them I'd eaten when in fact I hadn't, that I forced myself to vomit the meals they did see me eat. All they saw was a thinner me and that everything was fine on the outside.

I remember going to the Arab club on the weekends and at about 9:00 p.m., when my father sat down to play cards, he'd whistle to call me over. He'd ask, "Did you eat dinner?" When I said no, he told me to order something to eat. I remember ordering chicken with tabouleh, since it was the healthiest item on the menu. I also ordered toast, because I'd heard a rumor that if it was toasted, it was "lighter." Every crazy word-of-mouth suggestion I heard, I believed and applied to my makeshift diet. Even still, I was conflicted: *Is this going to make me gain weight?* Although I was dying to eat some French fries or dreamed how good a piece of baklava would taste, the constant fear of putting the weight back on was stronger than any craving. The fear was so great that it become a hazard to my health. But I hadn't realized it.

So I would order dinner at the club and when I got home at 11:00 p.m., I tried to go to the bathroom to throw up. Sometimes, there was something to throw up, others there wasn't. I'd end up feeling sick afterward. The whole process was so unpleasant. Throwing up made me dizzy. It was like being in a battle with my own body; I'd choke, tear up, my ears would plug up. I decided it would be easier to just lie. After that, when my father asked me if I'd eaten, I'd say yes, even though

I hadn't had anything since lunch. It seemed like the perfect solution. It got him off my back, and I didn't have to worry about gaining weight or having to vomit.

The truth is parents often don't find out what is happening with their teenager when their child is intent on hiding it. If you put on a brave face, they believe that everything is fine. In my case, the thinner they saw me, and the happier I was about my weight loss, the happier they were for me. They had no idea that I was beyond skinny, way below my ideal weight. Neither did I. I see pictures of myself from back then and I'm shocked at how skeletal I looked. But I can remember feeling that no matter how thin I was, I didn't see myself as thin. It was only when I was twenty-three that I started to see myself as slender. But I was a long way from there at sixteen, because as much as I had slimmed my body, I hadn't managed to lose my emotional weight. I didn't even know it existed.

After I lost all the weight that had been torturing me throughout my adolescence, food went from being my refuge to becoming my nemesis. I no longer saw it as nutrition, but as something that could harm me. That doesn't mean I didn't still love it. I'd satiate myself with pictures of food in cookbooks and magazines that looked so delicious, but couldn't affect me physically. Clearly, I was battling a severe eating disorder, but in my little town, there wasn't a lot of information about eating disorders, so I didn't know that any of this was bad for my health. I felt dizzy and weak, but the desire to keep the weight off was stronger. I wanted to continue wearing the skinny clothes and receiving all the attention for looking so good, but, thank God, one day my body said "enough is enough."

Coming home one afternoon, I got in the elevator and all of a sudden, everything went black. As I was collapsing, I must have reached out to steady myself and I grabbed on to the edge of the elevator mirror, which shattered into a million pieces and fell on top of me as I passed out. When the elevator doors opened, they found me on the floor, my hand covered in blood from a dozen cuts. The next thing I remember was waking up in my apartment, surrounded by the worried looks of my parents and sisters. For the first time, they realized something serious was happening to me.

They took me straight to our family doctor to have him look at my hand and to see if he could explain what was going on with me. I felt super weak. They ran a series of blood tests and the doctor inspected my bruises, which everyone now discovered. My body had been sending distress signals that I had managed to ignore until that moment. I was horrified as I listened to the doctor tell my parents that, according to the blood work, I was dehydrated, deficient in several key vitamins and nutrients, and anemic. This made him believe I might have cancer. He asked my parents to step out of the room so he could speak to me alone for a moment.

He started asking me a serious of questions, and with the word "cancer" still ringing in my ears, I decided to be completely honest. I knew something terrible was going on with my body and this was no time to pretend everything was fine. The word "cancer" had frightened me and I was willing to do whatever it took for this doctor to help me. I told him everything I had done to lose weight and keep myself skinny. I told him how I never ate in the morning, that I only had lunch, and that on nights when my family forced me to eat dinner, I'd go upstairs and throw up and come back down acting like nothing had happened. I told him I'd hidden all this from my parents and that until that day they had no idea there was anything wrong with me.

After a series of questions and hours of physical exams, the doctor came to me and gave me his diagnosis: "Alejandro, cancer isn't causing your symptoms. You have pre-anorexia and we have to treat this right away." He also explained that throwing up after eating is a symptom of bulimia. *Anorexia. Bulimia.* These were new words in my vocabulary. I'd never heard of either so I had no idea what they meant—but at least it wasn't cancer, I thought.

"We have to admit you," he said finally. When he said they needed me in the hospital to give me an IV to hydrate me and give me nutrients, I was scared—not because of having to be in the hospital, but because I was scared of gaining weight again. The doctor used my fear for my own good. He told me that if I didn't follow his orders, they'd only have to do it all over again, but the next time I'd probably have to spend *weeks* in the hospital away from my parents until they got me to a safe place. It seemed like a nightmare, and his tactics worked.

I spent the night in the hospital, and I promised to take all the supplements he gave me. The next several nights, my mother made sure that I ate all the chicken-and-potato soup she made to nourish me. I couldn't help thinking, *Ugh, this is going to make me gain weight*, but I figured it was better than having to go back to the hospital. I spent four weeks like this, following the doctor's guidelines to a T. Although I was scared of gaining weight, I continued to follow his orders and never went back to the bathroom to throw up.

I'd finally understood the gravity of the matter. I wanted to be healthy again, not just for me but to stop worrying my poor parents. After many years and many psychotherapy sessions, I realized that the problem was that I was still angry at the chubby little voice inside that had made me suffer so much; I hadn't made peace with him yet. I still didn't love who I was. I still needed to identify my emotional weight, to take stock of the emotions inside me. That's why I keep insisting that dealing with this is so important.

And that's how, about two or three weeks after my fainting spell, I came to find myself visiting psychologists, psychiatrists, and life coaches, trying to find a new path forward. I needed a way to open the doors to my emotions to identify the emotional weight that was flattening my spirit.

GET RID OF WHAT DOESN'T HELP YOU AND KEEP FORWARD ON YOUR PATH

When you begin to take stock of what you feel, when you face it down, that's when you finally start on the road to recovery and health. After identifying that pain, that emotional weight, you need an emotional detox to get rid of everything that doesn't help you, to stop being the victim of insecurity, to make room for the healthy version of you to develop inside and out.

Besides recognizing your emotional weight, it's important to recognize the external factors that can knock you off course.

Besides recognizing your emotional weight, it's important to recognize the external factors that can knock you off course. You can't allow anyone to make you feel bad. You have to learn to let go of others' aggression, manipulation, and guilt so they don't affect you on a personal level. I know it's not something you can do overnight. Something that has hurt you for so many years doesn't just stop hurting you in an instant. The goal is to make that pain, that person, that experience, affect you less and less over time. You can't let outside factors keep having power over you and your emotions. *You* have the power. And once you realize that, you'll see it becomes much easier to let go of things that used to make you feel powerless and heartbroken. You take the power away from the situation, and now *you* have control—and starting on this day, the power to live the life you want is solely in your hands.

At about eighteen or nineteen years old, after many therapy sessions and seminars, I finally understood why I turned to food. In my case, it was to substitute my parents' love. I ate to fill that void, to get attention, to ease my sadness and loneliness. And I learned that change had to start with me. Food had only made the situation worse, and even when I lost weight, I hadn't managed to pay attention to my inner self.

When you make such a major change in your life like losing weight, if you don't give yourself space to reflect on what's happened, you're going to have a disconnect between what you are and what you want to be. You have to make the inside consistent with the outside. Now that you've identified your emotional weight, it's time to leave behind the old coping tools, the ones you used to get attention or to shield yourself from pain. It's time to find new tools. You'll have to grow, evolve, learn to love and accept yourself, make peace with your past and connect with your present. It's time to reconnect with your deepest desires and focus on reaching your dreams. It's time to define your goals. Keep reading. I know you can accomplish it.

Essential advice to transform your life

- To change what's on the outside, you also have to change what's on the inside.
- Pay attention to how you behave with food.
- Think about what you're doing and what you're feeling when you turn to food when you're not actually hungry.
- Stop being your own worst enemy.
- Be conscious of your problem and your environment so you can make the necessary changes. Do it!

Put It into Practice!

YOU HAVE TO KNOW YOUR ENEMY TO DEFEAT HIM

When I was at my heaviest, I stopped looking in the mirror altogether. I didn't even want to see that obese person anymore. My reflection was trying to ask me for help; that person was clearly ignoring something much deeper than his weight. But I didn't recognize that image as my own. Instead, it was my worse enemy and I wanted to avoid my reflection at all costs. Now, I want you to do the opposite. Once and for all, I want you to look at yourself, to really *see* yourself, recognize yourself, rediscover yourself. Be honest with yourself so you can finally heal and love yourself.

Stand in front of the tallest mirror in your house, so you can see yourself from head to toe. Make sure you're alone, stripped down naked or to your underwear and nothing else. Look at yourself right in the eye—your eyes. Recognize those eyes. Observe them. Connect with your emotions and what they make you feel. Breathe: in through your nose, out through your mouth. Look at your eyebrows, your nose, your lips, your ears, your hair, your face. Connect with your emotions and be aware of what you feel. Lower your eyes and look at your body, your chest, your arms, your hands. Connect with your emotions and be aware of what you feel. Put your right hand over your heart. Breathe. Now look at your waist, your stomach, your legs, your feet. Connect with your emotions and be aware of what you feel. Breathe. As you run your eyes over your body, recognize where your fat is, how it looks, how it feels, how many little dimples and curves it has. Look at your skin, your scars. Breathe.

Now, on a piece of paper, write down what you feel, and how it feels to see yourself so clearly. What emotions surface? Are they pleasant or painful emotions? Write down the good as well as the bad. Congratulate yourself for doing it! It's not an easy exercise but it's essential before you can take the next steps toward healing yourself inside and out. Do it!

Dania Hernández

My name is Dania Hernández. I'm thirty years old, born in Guatemala but living in Rhode Island. When I was little, my parents abandoned me, and I was raised by my grandparents. I had a tough childhood, since my grandfather was an alcoholic. I had to endure my family's mistreatment and rejection. Trying to escape this life, I rushed out and got married at fifteen. I never imagined that my ex-husband also struggled with alcoholism. I was a victim of domestic violence for a long time. He would humiliate me, calling me fat, telling me nobody loved me, and that the only thing I was good at was eating.

My only trusted company, the only thing that never abandoned me, was food. It became my refuge, my answer for everything. I grew to weigh 235 pounds and developed Type 2 diabetes. The doctor told me, "Either you take care of yourself of you're going to die." I felt helpless.

I lost myself to addictions to both alcohol and food in order to forget my situation. I thought there was no hope until I met my angel Alejandro Chabán and his Yes You Can! *The supplements, nutrition, movement, and emotional health started transforming my life, burning all the fat in my body, face, arms, and belly.*

Yes You Can! *has given me back my health, my smile, and my desire to fight for my dreams. I've lost eighty pounds in nine months, to date. I dropped from a size 3XL to a medium. Today, I feel loved, supported by my* Yes You Can! *coaches and by my* Yes You Can! *family.*

SUCCESS STORY

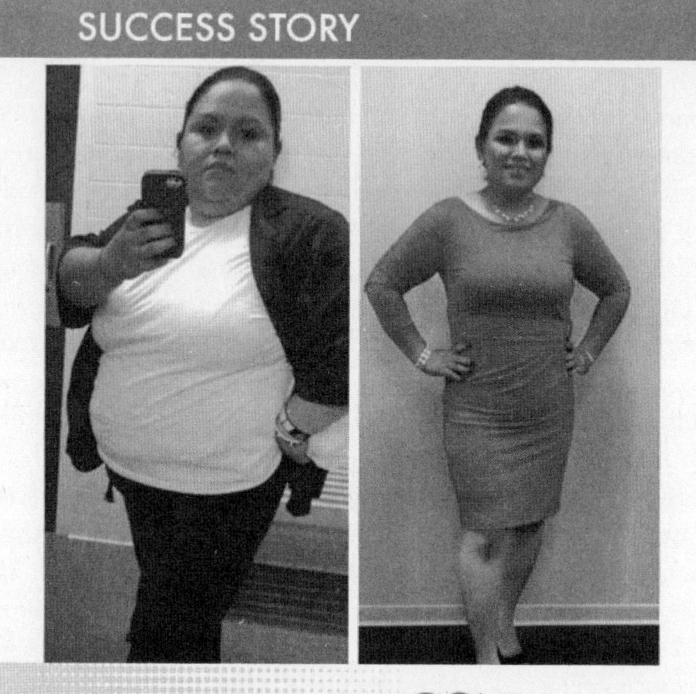

DANIA HERNÁNDEZ lost 80* lbs

DANIA'S ADVICE: *What helped me achieve change was documenting my journey on social media so I could see my progress and finding support within the Yes You Can! community. I had proof that I had made a change!*

**Results not typical and will vary according to diet, exercise, metabolism, and genetic makeup.*

(SIX)

Step 3: Set Your Goals

WHEN WE'RE IN the eye of the hurricane, surrounded by all this swirling extra physical and emotional weight, reaching our hopes and dreams can feel like such an uphill battle that it seems practically impossible. For me, at the time, being overweight was like having a life sentence. Losing 150 pounds seemed like such a distant and impossible goal that it was easier to just keep eating. I didn't even know where to start. I was lost and almost literally drowning in my fat.

It's as if someone tells you to walk from Los Angeles to New York—without a map. Are you kidding me? Where would you even begin? What if you got lost along the way? What if you didn't like what you found when you got there—if you got there? No, you'd think, it's better that I just stay in Los Angeles because I'm comfortable here and at least I know my surroundings. It's my comfort zone. It's my known universe. That's the same anxiety you feel when you have to lose so much weight, inside and out. You have no idea where to go, how to get there or if you'll even succeed. You don't know whether you're going to fail or die on the way there. This is where goals come into play, the essential step in attaining what you most want in life.

To establish a goal,
first you need to state your desire.

To establish a goal, first you need to state your desire, such as losing weight, buying a house, finding a new job. Then you turn that desire into a goal that's clear, realistic, and tangible, setting a deadline and writing out a projection plan—this will be your road map to achieving your dreams. Having clear, specific goals is the key to success in any endeavor. If you say you want to lose weight but you can't even say how much you weigh now, how many pounds you want to lose, and by when you want to lose them, then you don't have a clear goal and the task becomes much more difficult. How are you going to reach your destination if you don't even know how to get there?

Let's say, for example, you want to go to Disneyland. You hop in your car and head for the highway, but you have no idea when to turn. So you pull off and ask some random stranger how to get there. She says, as far as she can remember, that you should turn left at the next intersection and then take your first right. You follow her directions but you realize you're still lost. At the end of the block, you run into another person at the gas station and ask him for help. He says the directions the woman gave you are all wrong. He says you should make a U-turn and turn at the light. You do it, but you're still lost. You roll down the window and a truck driver says you should get off at the next exit. Keep that up and you'll be at this for hours before you ever reach your destination—if you reach it. You get frustrated and want to just turn around and go home. You don't even want to go to Disneyland anymore. You're in a bad mood and really hating this trip—until you notice the car has a GPS. You turn it on and first determine where you are. Then, you decide where you want to go, which will tell you how long it will take to get there, the possible routes, and the distance. You can now focus on the goal, thinking about how badly you want to go and how fun it will be when you get there. You'll focus on what's really important, which will help you visualize the trip and take the appropriate actions. Remember: A desire without a goal or a plan is only a dream. If you want to turn it into a goal, you have to determine your plan of action and set a date for completion.

> *A desire without a goal or a plan is only a dream.*

The point to this story is that you should never set off down a path someone else maps out for you because you could end up arriving later than you ever expected, if at all. You don't know whether this person made the trip in a car, bus, train, or on bicycle. You don't know whether they were in a rush or if someone else was driving. Get in your car, punch the address into your GPS, and decide on your course. As it relates to your diet, ask yourself, what diet should you follow? Do you like to cook and prepare food? Then you'd be a Food Lover Dieter on Yes You Can! Always on the road? Then you'd be an On the Go Dieter. If you decide to make the journey with someone at your side, make sure he or she supports and pushes you, and doesn't make you lose focus or fill your head with negativity. You have the power to decide your own course. The time has come for you to take the next step in your life toward reaching your dreams, healing your soul, and finding good health.

ESTABLISH CLEAR AND REALISTIC GOALS

It doesn't matter what your wish is, if you don't have a clear vision of what you want, how it will help you, the time it will take to achieve it and the necessary determination to reach it, then your goals are dead in the water. The reason you have to be so clear and specific about your goals is that otherwise what you get might not be what you want. Maybe you have a mental image of what you want. But it should be very specific. Otherwise, you may not be satisfied with the results.

It's like when you go to a restaurant. You don't sit down and ask the waiter to bring you food. You ask for the menu, read it calmly, look at all your options, check the prices, choose your dish, and then you are ready for the waiter. You tell him exactly what you want to eat, from the appetizer to the main course to dessert to coffee. That's exactly what you should do with your goals, too. Instead of saying, "My goal this year is to be happy," be specific. Make a list of the things that would make you happy, then focus on achieving those goals. The more clear, vivid, and detailed the goal, the easier it will be to achieve it in the long run.

The more clear, vivid, and detailed the goal, the easier it will be to achieve it in the long run.

Besides being clear and specific, your goals should be possible, attainable, tangible—realistic. You can't think you're going to become a millionaire selling air-conditioners to Alaskans. Get me? Being unrealistic can only lead to frustration. If you're four feet tall and decide your goal is to play basketball—or if you're seven feet tall and decide you want to be a jockey—I've got bad news for you: You're probably not going to be able to reach that goal because it's not realistic. You have to adjust your thinking.

Now, if you tell me you want to lose sixty pounds, that's definitely tangible and possible. But if you want to do it in an unrealistic amount of time, like in a week, that goal immediately becomes impossible. If you set an impossible goal, you're going to feel frustrated and you might even give up, thinking your effort is all for naught. But that's not how you do it! All you have to do is adjust the amount of time you'd set aside to achieve your goal. One week is unrealistic, but six months or a year are much more reachable. Don't you feel better knowing you've given yourself more time to reach your goal? And to reach that goal of losing sixty pounds in a year, you'll have to set other clear, specific, and real goals along your journey to reach your final destination.

THE THREE TYPES OF GOALS TO SUCCESS

There are three types of goals: short-term, medium-term, and long-term. You need all three working together to reach your ultimate goal. Your day-to-day, week-to-week, month-to-month goals all have to be in line with your ultimate goal so you can achieve it in the time you set out.

A short-term goal might be something you can achieve in one to three months. A medium-term goal might take six months to achieve. A long-term goal is one you hope to achieve at the end of a year. For example, if you're in high school and your goal is to go to college, your short-term goal is getting good grades. Your medium-term goal is passing each semester, and your long-term goal is getting into college. See how the short- and medium-term goals work hand in hand with the long-term goal? They're the key to achieving your dreams.

Perfect example: If you get out of bed one morning and decide you want to run a marathon, but you've never trained a day in your life, then that immediately becomes a long-term goal. If you try to make it a short-term goal, you're not going to meet it; you're going to be exhausted for having tried and then you will feel bad for having failed. But if you set it as a long-term goal, it becomes realistic and possible. So you have to ask yourself a set of questions to establish your short- and medium-term goals: Where can I train? How will I do it? Who can train me? How much time will I need to get ready? Each of these questions will help you figure out what you need to do to reach your long-term goal.

Another example: Say you want to land a job where you can make a million dollars. It's not an impossible goal, but it will take time and effort, so you have to make that a long-term goal. To figure out how much time you'll need to reach that goal, you have to evaluate your current position and try to determine which path you need to take. If you don't know anything about business, maybe you'll have to go back to college and study for a career in something that will net you a million dollars in a certain amount of time. As you can see, you have to ask yourself several questions and be as specific and realistic as possible. If you're telling me you want to be a millionaire, but you don't have a job, sleep until noon, and stay home watching television all day, well, then that goal isn't compatible with your way of life and you're not going to reach it.

Or let's say that, like many others, your goal is to own your own home. That would be your long-term goal. It's important to clearly define that goal so you can then set the medium- and short-term goals that will help you get there: Where do you want to buy a house? In what neighborhood? Do you want a house or a condo? What other amenities do you want in your home? Do you want to live in the city or the suburbs? How many bedrooms? One story or two? With or without a yard? Do you want to build your own? Define your goals clearly.

Once you've worked out the details of your long-term goal—in this case, your dream house—it's time to work on the medium-term goals. In this case, it could be a budget to help you save enough money to buy the house of your dreams. To meet that medium-term goal, you have to decide how much you can save a month—and how much you can give up spending every month in order to reach that goal. That's where your short-term goals come into play. Okay, so now you know how much you need to save a month, but say you don't have a job.

So the short-term goal becomes finding a job that allows you to save enough to buy the house of your dreams. Short-term goals serve as encouragement to keep you moving forward. It's amazing how rewarding it is to meet a goal, even a short-term one. It fuels you to keep going.

Put It into Practice!

SET REALISTIC GOALS

To make sure your long-term goal is realistic, ask yourself these questions:

- How long have you felt this way?
- How long have you been carrying around this excess baggage of toxic emotions and emotional weight?
- Do you also have physical weight that you want to lose?
- How much weight do you want to lose?
- What's your waist size?
- How much do you weigh right now?
- How much do you want to weigh?
- How much time do you want to or can you invest in your goal?

Remember: If you've been carrying around this emotional and physical weight for years, you can't expect to shed it in a couple of weeks. It's not a realistic goal. That's why all these questions are important. You have to take all of this into account to make a realistic goal. This way, you can heal your heart little by little, carefully, patiently, lovingly, respectfully. You can slowly begin losing the physical and emotional weight you're tired of carrying around and fulfill the commitment to yourself.

Make sure your short- and medium-term goals align with your long-term goals.

Make sure your short- and medium-term goals align with your long-term goals. When I lived in Los Angeles, I smoked a lot, up to two packs of cigarettes a day when I was having financial troubles. Even now, when I look out onto my balcony, I miss smoking a cigarette out in the breezy, open air. But I don't do it because I don't smoke anymore. I stopped the moment I decided my goal was to inspire millions of others to live a healthy lifestyle. That's when I realized my smoking habit wasn't aligned with my long-term goal of being a healthy person and a motivational figure. So I said to myself, "No more." I dumped the box into the sink and then tossed the squishy pack in the trash. If I wanted to inspire you to be healthy inside and out, I can't very well do the opposite and smoke. I'd be a hypocrite. I can't motivate you to improve your physical and emotional health if I'm addicted to nicotine. It's not in line with my long-term goals. You have to question your behaviors and actions and ensure that they align with your long-term goals. Is what you're doing today in step with where you want to be tomorrow?

If you want to heal your emotional weight, the two goals you have to have reach at this point in the book are: making a commitment to yourself and identifying your emotional weight to determine the root of your problem. Have you done it? Good! Congratulations! Take advantage of the satisfaction you're feeling at having met those short-term goals and use it as fuel to keep going. Short-, medium- and long-term goals are essential motivation so you won't give up on your final destination. It doesn't matter whether the goal is large or small. What's important is that it's important to *you*.

MY FIRST GOAL

My father was the person who helped me establish my first goal. It was one of the things that motivated me to lose weight. He told me, "C'mon, champ! You're strong. You have the fire and the power inside you to reach this goal!" It was that desire to lose weight—with my parents supporting me—that inspired me. To have them at my side, believing in me, and telling me all along that I could do it was my light at the end of the tunnel. The other was the motorcycle my dad promised me if I reached my goal.

He knew how much I wanted a little motorcycle. I dreamed about riding it to meet up with my friends in town. My dad turned that dream into a long-term goal when he came up to me one day. "I have an idea," he told me. "Let's make a deal: If you lose weight . . . I'll buy you that motorcycle." I was awestruck! Suddenly, that dream became something tangible, and my dad had shown me the way toward the goal. It was a huge motivation, the first concrete goal that kept me focused. Whenever I wanted to throw in the towel, when I was upset at not losing how much I'd hoped in a given week, the image of that motorcycle floated into my head and kept me from giving up. However, what kept me focused day to day was the sense of relief and lightness I started to feel as I lost weight. It also helped to hear the positive feedback from those who noticed I was thinner. The knowledge you could see physical changes, that my effort was paying off, was a huge inspiration to stay on track with my goals.

When I finally reached my ideal weight, my dad made good on his promise and bought me that motorcycle. He rewarded my efforts and I reached my long-term goal: losing all the weight, keeping the commitment to myself, and getting the motorcycle of my dreams!

Put It into Practice!

NOW IT'S YOUR TURN

Choose one of your goals and, as motivation, choose a prize you will give yourself upon reaching it. Make sure the prize has nothing to do with food. Instead, make sure it's something that inspires you, motivates you, something that you're passionate about and will make you happy. For example:

- If your goal is to drop twenty pounds and you love music, once you reach that goal, go buy a ticket to see your favorite artist in concert.
- If your goal is to submit your immigration documents so you can help your family, then when you reach your goal, throw a party to celebrate with your loved ones.
- If your goal is to get a new job and you love golf, when you get hired, treat yourself to golf lessons.

Having a reward waiting for you at the end of the road serves as a great motivator for reaching your destination. Remember, it doesn't have to be a big, lavish gift. It simply has to be something that will make you happy. Use it to celebrate your achievement!

WILLPOWER'S ROLE IN REACHING YOUR GOALS

As I fought to lose weight and later when I battled anorexia, I had to have an immense amount of willpower to overcome those challenges. Life is full of tempting impulses and if we let those impulses control the choices we make on our journey, we'll never be able to reach our goals. They will knock us off track. That's where willpower comes in. You can control those small impulses and behaviors so that you can reach your goal. That strength, that power, is within you. If your goal is to lose weight and someone offers you a slice of cake, you are the one who gets to decide if you fall off the wagon and eat the cake or whether you'll hold steadfast. That decision comes from your willpower. It's what helps us overcome the obstacles in our journey and keeps us heading toward our goals.

> *You can control those small impulses and behaviors so that you can reach your goal. That strength, that power is within you.*

You're probably asking yourself, "But where's my willpower? Where is it hiding? How do I tap into it when I need it?" When you find yourself in one of these situations, before answering, stop for a moment and think about your goal. If you take the slice of cake, will this help you reach your goal? No. So don't take it. I *know* you have the willpower to make the right decision. Now, all you need is to believe it yourself.

Do you know where your willpower is? Inside you! As a matter of fact, I think we're all born with the same amount of willpower. But as the years go by, some develop it and strengthen it more than others. Sometimes, life's circumstances dim it, or hide it. And those of us who lose sight of our willpower think we never had it at all. But we do, I promise you that. If you feel this way, you have to find out why you weren't able to develop and nurture your willpower.

- What habits or beliefs have blocked your willpower so badly that you have lost faith in your decision-making skills?
- What circumstances have made you feel like that power is no longer in your hands?

Many of us come from a different country. And sometimes, the daily struggle in a new country, from the language to the culture, can feel like such an insurmountable climb that we lose some of our willpower. Where did you leave it? It's always there, but you've just lost sight of it.

What helped me rediscover my willpower was setting goals. If I don't have a clear and specific goal and the desire to reach it, then I don't have the willpower to meet it. If there's not something to motivate and inspire me, I find I don't have the strength to talk down the chubby little voice inside me, and he can make me feel like a victim. But if I'm focused on something, there's no stopping me. If I know what my destination is, my willpower asserts itself so I can visualize my goal daily and achieve it. I know it's not easy sometimes and that it takes huge effort. But I also know that if you're determined, willpower fills you with energy and motivation and you feel like you can take on the world.

That's why it really bothers me when I hear someone say something like, "I'm single. Forty. Always been fat. I'm unhappy. No one loves me. I don't have any friends. But I can't stop drinking wine." Seriously? For a few glasses of wine a day you're giving up on all those other things you want in your life? Are you going to let a glass of wine, an order of French fries, or a plate of pasta get between you and your dream? That glass of wine isn't more important than your health or helping you build the family you desire. If you don't agree, I want you to go back and read this chapter from the beginning because clearly you haven't yet made a commitment to yourself. But if you do agree that a glass of wine or a French fry isn't more important than your happiness, then do this next exercise.

Put It into Practice!

DISCOVER YOUR WILLPOWER

If you had to rate your willpower today on a scale of 1 to 10, what number would it be? Think about it. Okay, have that number in mind? Well let me clear up something right now: We're all born with a 10! Get what I'm saying? If you answered any other number, I want you to make it a 10 in your mind right now. Maybe in the passing days, months, or years, you've lost sight of that 10, but it's been inside you all along! I want to plant that seed of willpower in your mind.

Now, plant that seed, along with the number 10, deep in your soul and water it every day so that it never dries up again and blooms into all the desires you deserve. How do you nurture your willpower? Every time you reach a milestone—whether that's exercising, not criticizing someone, sticking to your diet, landing a job interview, losing weight—no matter how small:

- Reflect for a moment over what you accomplished.
- Recognize the effort and decision you made to reach it.
- Smile!
- Pat yourself on the back!
- Congratulate yourself!

Celebrate each of these moments, and that way, your willpower will continue to grow.

YOUR PURPOSE IN LIFE

The first step you have to take to discover your purpose in life is to ask yourself the following questions. Please write your answers next to the questions. It's important for you to see your answers. Answer honestly. No one is going to judge you. You have to connect with your desires, dreams, and deepest passions. Dare yourself to smile:

- What's important to you in life?

____

- What motivates you to keep going?

____

- What would you dare to do with your life if you knew you couldn't fail?

____

- What dream have you always had but you never accomplished because you were scared or you thought you couldn't achieve it?

____

- What do you want out of your life?

____

- What do you want your legacy to be?

____

So often the things we want in life don't line up with what we're currently doing. You can ask some people what they really want out of life and they may say they want to have a family. But if you ask these same people what kind of car they want, they answer a two-door BMW. That doesn't go hand in hand with their supposed goal in life to have a family. That car won't easily fit a baby seat or a stroller because it's not a family car. If your goal is to start a family, the kind of car you are looking for should match that goal.

> *Your goals are directly related to your purpose in life. And this purpose will be revealed in the things you value.*

As you'll see, your goals are directly related to your purpose in life. And this purpose will be revealed in the things you value. Our purpose and goals in life are, and should be, completely personal. It's what sets us apart from the rest of the world. If you want to make money, fine. Travel the world, that's fine too. If your calling is to do works of charity, great! If you find your worth in a profession, more power to you! If your greatest desire is to meet someone and fall in love, excellent! Your purpose in life is yours alone. It's a very unique and personal path. It doesn't answer to obligations or debts. It's about your passion, your love, your inspiration, what makes you whole.

I know a brilliant guy, super intelligent and extremely capable. One day when his boss told him that he was being promoted to manager, he was firm in his answer: No. That position wasn't in line with his goals. He valued his free time, playing sports, and going out with his partner. He was fine with the salary he was making and he didn't want any more responsibilities. He knew what made him happy and focused on that. Your priorities don't make you a better or worse person. In fact, if we all had the same goals and purpose, how boring life would be! The beauty is that each one of us has our own dreams and each of those dreams complement someone else's dream. And that's the way the world comes together, each of us offering something unique and special. That's how we enrich one another. How marvelous!

Imagine if that friend of mine knew exactly what he wanted but he took on a great role because of societal or familial pressure. First of all, he would be trying to meet someone else's goal, not his. He would lose sight of his own goals, his own priorities, and that would probably make him feel sad or even depressed. What happens when we feel sad—when we gain emotional weight? We run to something that helps us fill that void—something like food. And that's where my friend's free fall would begin. By giving in to societal or familial pressures, he would lose sight of his own purpose in life.

Goals that are not aligned with our purpose bring unhappiness. We end up working toward something that, deep down, isn't what we want. That causes us frustration and resentment. What you're doing stops making sense. I could say to you, "You'll be a millionaire!" But maybe you'd answer, "Wait, that's not what I want." Right, so what is it that you want out of your life? More important, is your emotional or physical weight helping you reach that goal?

It's not about judgment. I'm not going to judge you. On the contrary, what I want most is for you to discover what makes you happy. Define your priorities, the things that are important to you. If what you want most is to get married, but your emotional and physical weight have isolated you from your friends, then clearly that's something you need to address. If you don't go out and socialize, you're never going to give yourself the opportunity to meet someone new, someone who would want to be with you. If being emotionally and physically overweight is preventing that, then that's the first stone you have to kick out of your path. How do you approach it? With short- and medium-term goals. You have to focus so you can identify your emotional weight. This will allow you to start losing your physical weight and healing your body and soul. That's the only path toward happiness.

IN SEARCH OF MY GOALS AND DREAMS

If we don't commit to ourselves and abide by the goals we set for ourselves, then we'll never be truly happy. As hard as it may seem, we have to follow our own path, find our purpose in life, and make it our priority.

Ever since I was eight years old, my dad has been preparing me to take over the business and run for governor of Maturín—which was his dream. Every morning when he drove me to school, he'd play motivational tapes, which had nothing to do with how I felt, but rather how he wanted me to be in the future. He set my short-, medium-, and long-term goals, but they were *his* goals, not mine. I was interested in the exact opposite of business at the time. I was interested in performing. It was a long-term goal I'd been developing ever since I was a child.

While my dad played those tapes and drilled into me that I would take over for him, run the store, and take care of my sisters, I was dreaming of something bigger—something that would take me far away from our little town. My family's daily routine in Maturín wore me down. I didn't understand why we couldn't do something different on the weekends. I wished that instead of taking our Sunday drive around town, which culminated with our stop at the ice cream shop, we could instead go to the river or have a picnic or head to the park or even church—anything to break the boring routine. But no.

Nevertheless, when I think back on this, I considered myself a happy child. I was calm, studious, and I wasn't at all difficult. Come to think of it, I was much more mature than other kids my age. I'd watch all the trouble others got into and would think to myself: *Why are they bothering that poor lady who's probably tired after a long day at work?* I'd even try to dissuade them, but that resulted in the other kids making fun of me and telling me they wouldn't play with me if I kept it up. It's when I first started feeling out of place.

Our place in the world isn't necessarily the spot where we're born. I didn't understand that until much later. Back then, as a quiet and sensitive kid, I didn't understand why I felt like I didn't belong. I remember lying under the stars at night wondering if other people, in other cities and other countries, were looking up at the same stars as me. I was very curious. I felt a calling to be something different. I think that's why I gravitated toward acting from the time I was young. It was an escape. I could pretend to live other lives, in other worlds, through my imagination. It was fascinating to me.

I remember a lot of my Arab friends were content to imagine themselves taking over the family business, happy to know they would one day work with their parents at their stores, and then, one day, it would be theirs. They didn't think it was boring to do the same thing every day, open and close the store at the same time, have the same lunches and dinners, never wondering what else life might have in store. Now, of course, I understand that was their choice. Doing that is what made them happy. That was their purpose in life, but it definitely wasn't mine. Which is why when I saw I might have the chance to leave Maturín and become a professional actor, I didn't hesitate.

It was June 1998 and I was about to graduate from high school when my father approached me with a plan.

"I want you to stay in Maturín for a year and then we'll figure out what to do next," he said.

"No," I told him flatly. "I'm going to college in Caracas and I'm leaving in August."

"But it's already June."

"It doesn't matter. I plan to leave in August."

I knew my dad didn't like the idea of letting me go off to the capital all by myself. Remember, I had skipped two grades. I was graduating from high school at sixteen and would be turning seventeen in August, right around the time I'd be arriving in Caracas. Nevertheless, my dad never stood in my way. He heard the determination in my voice and respected my desires. Now it was a matter of choosing a major. He asked the psychologist to help me pick a career.

Since I hated science and math, I wanted a career that had nothing to do with either of those subjects. To make sure of that, when I took vocational tests with the psychologist, I would do poorly on the science and math section on purpose to manipulate the results. But since I was someone who always loved to study, I thought that the best career for me might be law, so that's what I aimed for when taking the test. However, this choice was based on what would best fulfill my parents' wishes. That's all I wanted from my vocational test results because my short-term plan was just to get to Caracas, one way or another. And once there I would redefine my goals in order to become an actor. I had my path mapped out. Now, I just needed a way to bring it into being. Nothing was going to hold me back. Those goals had lit a fire inside me. All my willpower was directed at fulfilling what I felt was my greatest dream in life: acting.

Nevertheless, this dream of acting wasn't something I could talk about at home. They never took it seriously. Moreover, the word "actor" in my house was linked to drugs, vices, alcohol, and people who led an out-of-control life. No son of my father was ever going to live that kind of life. He needed me to have a traditional path while I wanted to go off to Caracas to fulfill my dream. So I used the most powerful and valuable tool I had at my disposal: my psychologist.

Once we decided that I would study law, in my sessions with him, I started mentioning how important it was for my mental state for me to leave Maturín. In previous sessions, I hadn't really opened up. But now I began speaking more frankly, in hopes that he would help me convince my father that moving to Caracas was for my own good. He understood how suffocated I felt. He understood how I suffered because I did not fit in and that staying home was the equivalent of a prison sentence. I needed to fly off toward something new, to a place where I could explore who this new and slender person was, someone who now was open to new hopes and possibilities.

My father heeded the psychologist's recommendations, and two weeks after graduation, we were in Caracas, touring the universities. I registered at a private university, where I could begin classes in the fall, and my father agreed to pay for everything. My father had some Maturín friends in Caracas who had an apartment and he rented it for me. And that's how I fulfilled my long-term goal of moving to Caracas, which was also a short-term goal in my dream of becoming an actor.

YOUR FUTURE IS IN YOUR HANDS

Now that you have your goals written down, remember to love yourself and congratulate yourself when you meet them. Each goal met is an achievement and it should be celebrated. What happens after you meet a goal? Celebrate, then make a new list of goals! Goals, just like the seasons, change and evolve over time. As we grow, we need other things in our lives. That's why we have to pay attention to our circumstances and readjust our goals accordingly. That way, our goals will always be aligned with our lives.

For example, when my last relationship ended, my life took another turn. It changed and I had two options: Either I locked myself in my house and slept, turning off the phone and crying, allowing myself to be a victim, or I could use the opportunity to grow, to take care of my health, and to improve my life. The first option wasn't going to solve anything. It wasn't going to bring back my lost love. And it was a path that could easily lead me back to using food as a comfort. So I chose the second option. I focused on my well-being and taking care of myself. Taking care of my body, my nutrition, my mind, and my soul. I had to stop and think about the consequences of my actions to reach that decision. When I face an emotional and painful event in my life, I ask myself, *Is what you're going to do next going to improve or resolve what you're feeling today?* If my answer is no, I look for another path. I reevaluate my goals and I pay attention to the new desires that arise from this moment. I think about what will fill my heart and soul with richness, and that is what will lead me to take care of my mind and spirit.

Another realization that can make you reevaluate your goals is when you discover you've set goals for the wrong outcome. When you realize that the thing you thought would make you happy doesn't really turn out that way. This is another moment when you should stop, pay attention to what isn't working, and reevaluate the path you're on. It happened to me with acting. When my first television roles started to air, instead of celebrating the moment, I was focused on something else. I thought, *Wow, when everyone who used to make fun of me sees how famous I am, they're going to have to eat their words and want to be my friends.*

And that's exactly what happened. The ones who had made the most fun of me now wanted to be my friends on Facebook, and I accepted a couple of them so they could witness my success—so I could show them I was more than they thought I was. But soon, it didn't have the same effect on my life. It's like when you save for three months to buy yourself those designer jeans or that new purse and you finally buy it and wear it with pride. And everyone at work tells you how great you look. But after the third or fourth day, the novelty wears off. The fact that those who used to make fun of me could see my success did nothing to erase the torment they had caused me emotionally. It didn't help reduce the pain I carried inside. Today, I realize that I had chosen a path linked with attention and approval, the things I'd longed for as a child. I thought this path would fill the void from the suffering I'd endured. But the only thing that could heal my pain was healing my emotional weight.

Meanwhile, the chubby little boy inside me continued looking for acknowledgment and love. He was still very insecure and filled with fears despite the fact that to others, on the outside, I seemed to be so put together. Now I realize that even our career path, our vocation, our calling, is linked to our childhoods. Back then, I hadn't realized what the purpose of my life was. I was thin and acting professionally. I'd reached all my goals. But it was time to make new goals. And to do that, I had to ask myself more questions. The first one being: What do I want to dedicate my life to?

Losing weight is only the first step toward accomplishing our higher goals. It is also important to heal our toxic emotions and our spirit. Because if we're beautiful on the outside but destroyed on the inside, we'll never be able to focus on the most important things in life—our dreams, our desires, our goals—with a clear purpose. But hold on tight, because when your mind, body, and spirit are united behind one cause, there's nothing you can't do!

I know that the reason I've been able to continue reaching my goals is because I've dedicated a lot of time and effort into healing my emotions. Without doing that, I could have never moved forward. We all have injuries in our past. In my case, it was rooted in my weight gain; for you, it might be something else. But what's clear is that if we don't heal ourselves, it won't be possible to keep moving forward and reaching the stars.

It's something I'm still working on today. I know I have certain emotional blocks that I have to uncover to keep striving toward my goals. I know now that the injured, overweight little boy who didn't think he was worth anything could never have reached such goals as having an international company, helping millions of people transform their lives, and making millions of dollars if he did not heal himself first.

Challenges are life's gifts to us,
because they help us grow.

We have to grow in life to learn how to handle new challenges that come our way. Challenges are life's gifts to us, because they help us grow. They are the surprises that give us an opportunity to improve ourselves so we can learn how to achieve our greatest desires. Without challenges, there are no valuable lessons in life. You have to fall so you can learn to stand back up. It's no fun, but that kind of learning comes only from experience. It's that simple. The way to keep those bumps from keeping you down is to set visible, reachable goals. Remembering that you achieved those goals helps keep you going down the path instead of sliding back. For example, once I'd started acting and aspired to reach the highest platforms at Univision, I'd think about my goals whenever I was tempted with food. I'd remind myself of the path I'd chosen and why. If I found refuge in food, I might gain back the weight, and then I'd never be a television star. That way of thinking is what fed my willpower so I could say no to temptation. And that's what I hope for you.

You are the architect of your own future.

It's not an easy road. Reaching our goals often requires great effort and sacrifice. But if you focus on your dreams, on your long-term goals, you'll remember that everything you're doing is in service of reaching your final destination. You are the architect of your own future. When you're on track, reaching your goals, approaching your dreams, then you'll be able to say you're living your dream life—the life that makes you happy. But to reach that point you're still missing some important steps. At this point in the book, you've already made a commitment to yourself. You've identified the root of your problems. And you've set your goals to reach your dreams, which will help reveal your purpose in life. Now you must learn to make affirmations that will help to reinforce these first three steps. Congratulate yourself. Love yourself. Celebrate and keep going! You're on the right track. Don't let anyone hold you back!

Essential advice to help transform your life

- Set clear, realistic goals. The more vivid and detailed they are, the easier they will be to achieve.
- Set short-, medium-, and long-term goals.
- Reconnect with your willpower. It's essential to reaching your goals.
- Discover your purpose in life. Remember that it should be directly related to your goals, values, desires, and passion.
- Celebrate each goal you achieve, then make new goals to keep moving forward with your purpose in life.

Put It into Practice!

DEFINE YOUR GOALS

Setting a goal is a strategy to help you reach your objectives and dreams. Now that you know how to set your own goals, it's time for you to write them down. Grab a pen and paper, open up your notebook or a new file on your computer, and write "My Goals" at the top. Now follow the next three steps to define them:

1. Write down your long-term goal, the desire or dream you wish to accomplish.
   - Make sure to be clear, specific, and realistic. This goal has to be consistent with your life.

- It has to be your goal and no one else's. There's no point in writing down your husband's or your children's or your parents' goals for you. You're making your story and yours alone.
- Write down a date. A goal without a deadline is just a desire. Write down the day, month, and year by which you'd like to achieve your goal. Be realistic with the time frame.

2. Now write down your medium-term goals, the ones you need to accomplish before reaching your final destination. Write down deadlines.
3. Lastly, write down your short-term goals, the things you have to accomplish today, tomorrow, next week, or next month so that you can take the next step forward. This will help you feel closer to your ultimate goal. Write down a deadline.

You may have more than one long-term goal. So simply repeat this process for each goal you have, whether it's buying a car, moving into a new house, changing jobs, starting a family, or going on a trip. Don't limit yourself. Being realistic doesn't mean you shouldn't think big. It begins today, right now, at this very moment. Doesn't matter what your goal is. The key is to maintain the desire in order to reach the end result.

Nidia Gámez

My name is Nidia Gámez and I'm twenty-seven years old. I'm the American-born daughter of Mexican parents. In my house, we always celebrated achievements with food. But I was always really skinny, so my mother used to give me vitamins to increase my appetite. I guess it worked because I started eating and after that I never stopped.

At age twelve, I was the victim of sexual abuse. I became depressed and locked myself in my room, eating out of control so I would make myself heavy. I wanted to be fat and ugly so no man would ever look at me again. I had low self-esteem because of the weight gain and my abuse. For years, I was embarrassed to go out and be seen at 216 pounds. And when I visited my family in Mexico, all I heard from my family was "You're so heavy, mija!*"*

*I finished high school, got married, and became a mother at a very young age. Although I had a lot of good things in my life, I was no longer Nidia. People just called me "*Gorda*" as a term of endearment in the Latin culture, but the word cut into me and depressed me. It made me eat more and more until I was a size XXL.*

Last year, tired of being called "fatty" as a nickname, I saw myself in a picture and noticed all the folds of skin. I realized that's how everyone saw me. I said, "Enough is enough." I started looking on social media for something that would help me lose weight and I discovered Alejandro Chabán, the angel who helped me reach my dreams.

I started with small goals, and in six months, I lost sixty-two pounds. Thanks to Yes You Can!, I feel like a new person, sure of myself, beautiful, and filled with big dreams. Yes You Can!

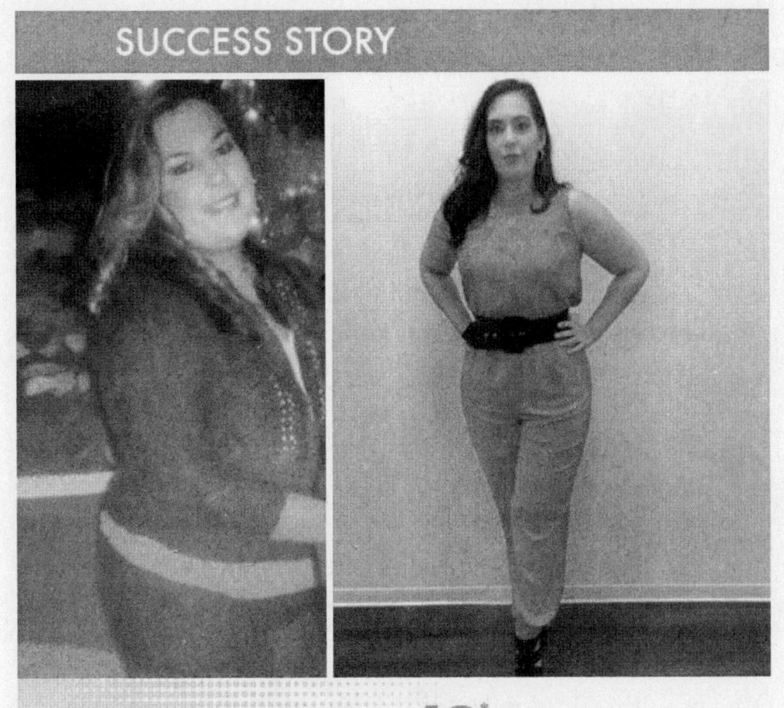

NIDIA'S ADVICE: *What helped me achieve these changes was setting small goals of losing five pounds at a time, instead of focusing on my huge, final number, which was my long-term goal.*

**Results not typical and will vary according to diet, exercise, metabolism, and genetic makeup.*

(SEVEN)

Step 4: Affirm Your Well-Being

WORDS ARE THE most powerful tools we have as humans. We can command armies with them. We can bring joy—and destruction. It's white magic or dark magic, depending on how we use it. Words are a gift from God. Words express your creative abilities. It is thanks to words that you can manifest what you dream, what you feel, and who you really are. With them you can create the most beautiful surroundings or destroy everything around you. You can even change your way of thinking just with words and you can accomplish this through affirmations.

I first learned about affirmations during a seminar in Venezuela. I was a bit lost on the inside at the time. Yes, I'd lost weight, had seen a psychologist, had started to identify my emotional weight, and had even moved to the big city to chase my dreams. But mentally, I still felt like I was that 314-pound kid. I was completely in limbo. I was a skinny person who thought he was obese, a young man who had moved to the capital to study law, while actually wanting to be an actor. At the same time, this new life offered me a blank page, a fresh start to write my own history, a play where I was the star. I needed to begin this new phase as the person I'd always wanted to be instead of the one who had made me suffer so greatly.

This was my big chance. Nobody knew my story. No one

knew what I had overcome in Maturín. No one knew how fat I'd been. It was the ideal time to transform myself, but I needed help. That's when affirmations came into my life, like a gift from above. They helped me begin the mental change I so wanted and needed to continue down the right path.

An affirmation is a sentence that aligns you with the future you desire.

An affirmation is a simple, positive sentence. This sentence aligns you with the future you desire; the power of these words can align you with your goal and help you reach a potential that you haven't yet discovered. An affirmation is a bridge between the person you are today and the person you aspire to be in the future. And just like any bridge, to cross from one side to the other takes more than good intentions. That's why your affirmations are so tied to your goals.

Just like goals, your affirmations have to be rooted in reality, too. If you repeat to yourself, "I have long, straight hair," but you were born with curly hair, it's not going to help you change your DNA. Similarly, you can't affirm something for someone else. If you begin saying to yourself, "My daughter *will* be an attorney," you'll soon realize that has nothing to do with you and everything to do with her. Affirmations, just like goals, have to be completely personal. It's part of that commitment to yourself and it comes from the goals you want to accomplish. Take a moment right now to look at your list of goals, the one you created in the previous chapter. Read it back to yourself slowly and consider what might keep you from achieving these goals. Now, think about the things that will help you achieve each goal on your list. This is the seed of your affirmation.

HOW TO MAKE AN AFFIRMATION

Affirmations have to be personal and positive. They have to refer to your ultimate goal and they have to be stated in the present tense. But to arrive at your affirmation, first you have to identify what you want to change about yourself. In the left-hand column of a piece of paper, write down a list of personal characteristics that you feel play against you. Those are your negatives. For example:

- Reclusive
- Unapproachable
- Fearful
- Sad
- Fat
- Insecure

Now, in the right-hand column, next to each word, write the opposite, what you would like to be versus what you think you are. Using the example above:

- Reclusive *Friendly*
- Unapproachable *Inviting*
- Fearful *Brave*
- Sad *Joyful*
- Fat *Slender*
- Insecure *Confident*

This exercise will help guide you in making your affirmation, a sentence that will serve as your daily mantra. From the list of positive words, pick three, four, or five and use them to focus on the change you want to see in yourself today. From our example, let's choose Brave, Joyful, Confident, and Slender.

Once you've chosen your own positive words, you have to compose a sentence using the words "I am." This will ensure that your affirmation will refer to your ultimate goal and not to the process that will take you there. This is the part that often confuses people. Often when I talk about affirmations, people don't pay attention and begin their affirmations with something like, "I wish . . ." But this has nothing to do with wishes. If you use a wish as an affirmation, then that's all it will ever be: a wish. And you will never be able to reach it. Others say, "Okay, well, then, how about 'I want . . .'" That's not right, either. If you affirm what you "want," you're always going to want something without doing what you have to do to get it. By starting your affirmation with "I am," it forces you to start becoming the person you want to be through your thoughts and actions. That's why you should start all your affirmations with "I am . . ." and always in the present tense to emphasize that your end result begins right now, in the present.

Another key to creating your affirmation is avoiding the words "no" or "not." Aside from the fact we want to keep the sentence positive, your brain doesn't recognize the word "no," even though intellectually you know what it means. If you say, "I am not fat," your brain doesn't recognize the word "no" and only focuses on the phrase "am fat." In this case, instead of saying, "I am not fat," you would say, "I am slender."

Words are more powerful than you think, so be careful what you choose as an affirmation. Make sure it reflects your goals. The idea is to *reaffirm* what you want. When I went to my first seminar in Caracas, years ago, not only did I learn what an affirmation was, but I followed the instructions and succeeded in creating my first-ever affirmation: "I am a humble and secure man, patiently healing my body in the universe." In this case, I chose the word "secure" because it is what I wanted to feel. Because even though I had lost 150 pounds, my mind was still that of someone who weighed 314 pounds. I chose the word "humble" because I felt the whole world was out to get me and I had become overly defensive. I chose "healing my body" because I had been obese and anorexic and I wanted to be a healthy person. I added "patiently" because I knew I had to be patient about healing my mind and body. I couldn't allow myself to become desperate. That's what had made me gain physical and emotional weight over the years. I couldn't very well change that overnight.

I want you to notice how detailed my explanation is for my affirmation. To this day, I can remember why I chose each word. And that's possible because I took my time to search deep within myself to find the words that would help me become the person I wanted to be. You have to take this step calmly. It's the time to explore who you are and who you want to be, a time to be honest with yourself, to look over your goals and open yourself to the possibility of reaching them.

HOW TO DEAL WITH NEGATIVE THOUGHTS

As we established in the beginning of this chapter, words are the most powerful instrument a human can possess. We can choose positive words that encourage or negative ones that destroy. Words hold the power to help, heal, block, damage, judge, criticize, gossip, and humiliate. The power vested in each word depends totally on you. That's why it's incredibly important for you to start paying more attention to your thoughts and actions. You have to stop the negativity before it takes over your thoughts and transform it into positive energy.

> *You have to stop the negativity before it takes over your thoughts and transform it into positive energy.*

During my weight-loss process, when I realized the reasons behind my voracious appetite—that I was compensating for my parents' affection—I started being conscious of my actions and paying closer attention to my daily behavior. That's what allowed me to change the negative conduct that was sabotaging me into new, uplifting, positive, and lasting habits. We'll explore that further in Chapter 9.

When you have negative thoughts, you will not be able to just blink them away on your first try. The most effective tactic is to tell your brain, "Thank you for your input," and turn back to your affirmation and goals. Those negative thoughts are like fears, expectations, or temptations: They never disappear completely, but you can learn to control them. Picture them like trees passing by your window as you drive down the road. If simply trying to refocus on your affirmation doesn't work, write down those negative thoughts, those fears, the feelings that paralyze you and keep you from your goals. The act of writing them down transfers them from your mind into something tangible; they become changeable. Now try repeating your affirmation, reread your goals, refocus on your intention, and shake off that negative energy. Adopt an active and positive attitude toward the changes you want to make in your life. Remember: Affirmations can be powerful and their energy can be either positive or negative. *It all depends on you.*

REAFFIRMING THE NEW YOU

I moved to Caracas at a time of personal discovery. I knew who I'd been in Maturín and I had an idea of who I wanted to be in the future. But my present was cloudy. That's why I decided to sign up for a personal growth seminar entitled *Insight*, which lasted four days. I'd heard about this organization some five years prior when my mother signed me up for an *Insight for Kids* seminar. At the time I was overweight and entering my rebellious stage. And since it was my parents' decision and not mine, I didn't know enough to take advantage of the valuable tools they were teaching me. It was so bad that one day my mother got a call to come pick me up. When she arrived, they told her I was too rude and my poor attitude was hurting the other children, who actually were ready to participate and learn.

They were right. I thought I was better than everyone else

and I was rude to the facilitators who were our guides. My mom didn't know how to handle all this. She didn't understand how I could be so good at my studies but be so rude to the rest of the world, including the teachers. She did everything she could to help me, but because I was not ready to accept help, the information went in one ear and out the other. And that's how it was with the seminar. Nevertheless, when I left for Caracas, my mother suggested the seminar again, and this time I was ready.

I arrived in Caracas feeling like the most insecure, reserved, sad, and lonely person in the city. I hated the world and felt the world rejected me in turn. My emotional health was lagging and I knew I needed help. Still, the fact that I'd lost all that weight gave me a feeling that I could conquer any obstacle in my path. I still needed to shed my emotional weight, but I was better prepared to confront the pain and fear I'd been avoiding all those years.

I took two *Insight* seminars in a span of two weeks. Those seminars are among the most amazing experiences of my life. I went in with the hope that they would help me recover my confidence and self-esteem. I wanted to learn to speak, dress, and act like a secure person. I wanted to feel like I finally belonged after years of feeling like an outsider. I wanted to finally become the healthy and slim person I was only beginning to discover. I came out of those seminars with my mind more open than ever. It was the beginning of the end of my emotional weight, an experience for which I will be eternally grateful to *Insight* and to my parents, who had the vision to realize what I needed most at that moment.

I experienced five intense, super-emotional days in which we all cried as we opened up and shared our deepest feelings, emotions that many of us never realized we had buried deep for so long. They helped us understand the root of these emotions. There were exercises to connect us to our inner child, what I like to call my inner chubby kid. They spoke to us in a familiar, soothing language. It reminded me of the tapes my dad used to play as he drove me to school in the mornings. It's where I learned to forget the word "no," because the mind doesn't recognize that word. It's where I learned what an affirmation is, where I learned to make my first affirming phrase, and where I learned what a vision board is. (We'll explore that further in the next chapter.)

That experience not only gave me endless new tools, many of which I still use today, but it also cleared up many things for me and helped me realize it was time to decide what things I wanted in my life and what I didn't.

At the end of the seminar, our emotions were so raw and fresh that the facilitators warned us not to make any huge or drastic decisions in the next few days, until everything settled down and we weren't quite so sensitive.

Just two weeks later, I started law school, which allowed me to absorb everything I had learned. I felt like many people in one body. I was the one who'd lost weight, the one who was beginning to affirm things I didn't yet feel, the one who had the tools but still felt insecure. But I had opened an important channel to my inner self. I spent the daily bus ride to school quietly repeating my affirmation to myself. I carried around my Discman so I could hear my motivational CDs by Camilo Cruz, Carlos Fraga, and Anthony Robbins during my downtime. They now inspired me and made me feel better.

Meanwhile, I stuck to my diet. I wasn't eating great yet, but I had learned to eat three meals a day, although sometimes I skipped dinner. Thank God, in Caracas there was more information and, for the first time, I was exposed to trainers and nutritionists, which really caught my attention. With school under control, I was able to make friends and found the time and space to focus on my next step, on my next goal, and that was tightening up my body—one of the only things that remained after losing all my weight. I was thin, but not at all toned. I needed to fix this and now I had the mental space to focus on it and achieve it. Plus, in Caracas it became more obvious because there were new fashion styles and I kept turning down my friends' invitations to go to the beach. No one knew about my past obesity and I didn't want them ever to find out.

As I'd mentioned earlier, although I'd dropped to a size small in my shirts with a 28- or 30-inch waist, I still had a flabby chest, stretch marks, and had no muscle tone whatsoever. So I got to work at finding information about it. Now my goal was to tone my muscles to see if that would fix my flabbiness. I started meeting trainers and nutritionists at the gym. I was open to all their advice and soon I started to see a difference. With exercise and nutritional supplements, I soon started to see visible results. I absorbed all their advice like a sponge. And I put all of it to the test to see what worked and what didn't. I remember going to school with a Tupperware full of hard-boiled eggs, and when I opened it, my classmates would say, "Ugh, that smells horrible!" But I no longer took those comments personally. I was super focused. If my trainer or nutritionist said I had to eat at a certain time, I did, without fail. I was super disciplined. I was doing everything I could to make my affirmations a reality.

When I started feeling more secure and was working to improve my physique, I turned my attention toward my true passion: acting. Five or six months had gone by and I had finished my first semester of college when I started finding out which acting classes I could take. When my father sent me the money to pay for the next semester, I didn't hesitate: Instead of paying for college, I used the money to pay for acting classes.

From that moment on, my focus changed completely. I'd arrive to acting class with my underlined scripts instead of my law books and I was so happy. I started to discover what it meant to follow your heart and do something that you're truly passionate about. The sensation is unrivaled. I could spend eight hours in acting class without even noticing, while in my law classes I was ready to run out screaming after an hour or two. When I was studying law, I felt tied down with obligation to my father. But in acting, I felt free. It fueled my spirit to keep up with acting and reaching for my goals.

As you can imagine, when my father found out I'd been using my school money for acting classes, he was seriously upset. He drove to Caracas, took me back to Maturín, locked me in my room, and told me if I didn't start behaving, I'd never be allowed out. But things had changed, and now nothing was going to hold me back. I knew my dream of being an actor was within my reach and no room or punishment was going to keep me from it. I wasn't going to sit still in that room for one more day. That's what inspired me to write him a letter, leave it on my nightstand, and escape out the window.

In the letter, I wrote that I had decided to return to Caracas to continue studying acting. I told him that no one had told him what he had to do with his life, that he had decided to follow his own desires. And similarly, it was my turn to find my own path and write my own story. And that's how I returned to Caracas. I moved in with a friend and my family didn't hear from me for months. I was so sure about what I wanted to do that I barely felt the anguish of cutting the cord to my family. Caracas to me signified freedom, independence. It was a breath of fresh air after feeling suffocated in a place where I felt I didn't belong.

When I turned eighteen, I withdrew the money I had in a savings account and bought swimsuits at a local factory, which I sold at school to make money. Since I'd cut ties with my family, I obviously wasn't receiving any money from them, so I needed some kind of income to survive. Moreover, when I left my parents the note, I also left them my cell phone, credit card, and the keys to the apartment. I needed to make a clean break. I lived off the money I made selling swimsuits and kept on with my plan.

Later I learned that when my family found my note, they were so worried. They spent weeks looking for me, until my father found my best friend's mother and she told him I was living with my friend in Caracas. At least they knew I was okay.

Months later, when they finally found me, they were more willing to hear me out. They wanted to know why I had made such a decision and gone against their will. Why I'd followed my path instead of preparing to take over the business. In the end, my parents signed up for an *Insight* seminar. I was so happy to be close to them again and that they were interested in bettering themselves as well.

After months of studying and endless auditions, I landed my first role on a *telenovela;* I was more determined than ever to follow a career in acting. My philosophy had always been to follow in the footsteps of the best actors, the people I admired the most. So I found out where the best Venezuelan actors studied or worked and went there. I started studying under an Argentine named Carlos Ospino and Nelson Ortega. I also got in with a television network, which sent me to a casting, and I landed my first role. In my second *telenovela*, I landed a leading role and that's when my career really started taking off. I couldn't believe it! My dreams were coming true!

Another goal reached! But as with all accomplished goals, there should always be a new one to take its place. Now, the pressure wasn't just to be thin and healthy, but to have the physique of a television actor like the ones I'd idolized in magazines since I was young. The time had come to turn my body into that of a leading man.

I figured out who trained the actors with the best physiques and I signed up to get his help. He recommended some great books and guided me so I would start to see food as nourishment and fuel for my body. I worked hard at cardio. And, being the good student that I was, I read all the books he'd recommended and fell in love with everything I was learning. It was fascinating to learn how nutrition affected the body, which foods did what, where the body stored fat and why, and which foods did what to affect my physique. A whole new world was opening up to me. Little did I know how important it would be to my career and to my purpose in life.

I trained with uncommon focus for months, following my diet to a T and following all my exercises. After a while, I made an important decision to reach my ultimate goal: gynecomastia surgery. The doctors removed the excess fat that had remained in my chest after I'd lost all my weight and they removed the excess skin. I'd spent the last four years wearing sweaters to cover my flabbiness. Looking at myself in the mirror and not seeing all that excess skin was another dream fulfilled—and yet another feeling of freedom.

After that, I started to really develop my muscles: my arms, my chest, my legs, my abs. It was still hard to believe that my body, which had once been obese, now had muscles and ripped abs. I was still surprised at seeing my defined physique. It was mine, but I still couldn't believe it.

Once I had the toned body of my dreams, I decided to have some pictures taken, and that's when I realized I still had a lot of work to do. I was more cut than ever, had impressive muscles, but my eye was still drawn to problem areas such as my belly button, my stretch marks, my hidden cellulite, the dark spots on my skin. I thought: *Look how sad my belly button looks. Look at the fat here, the stretch marks there.* I didn't allow myself to see how good I looked. I kept looking for flaws, imperfections, focusing only on that.

I was still living in the past. I felt that I had to improve more and more and more. Even when I had a rock-hard body, I still wouldn't walk down the street without my sweater on. I still carried it with me everywhere I went. My body was much further developed than my mind or my emotions. I had spent so much time focusing on my body, that I had neglected to pay attention to my emotions. I had grown some when I arrived in Caracas, opening a path to my inner self. But I let myself get distracted. I still had a lot of emotional weight to deal with. My moment would arrive, but I had to keep working on my goals, my affirmations, and my willpower.

ADJUST YOUR AFFIRMATIONS TO EVERY STAGE OF YOUR LIFE

From the moment I made that first affirmation in Caracas, I continued to make new ones. You can always adjust your affirmations as you grow and change. Once you achieve your affirmation, revise it according to what you want to accomplish next. I change my affirmations when I feel I'm repeating something that I already accomplished. For example, my affirmations today have nothing to do with losing weight, because it's something I feel I have control over. I also change them whenever I get too comfortable with an affirmation to the point where I'm even too lazy to repeat it. I know I am no longer connecting to it. That's when I stop and try to refocus. I think about the goals I have in the next few months. I think about where I am and where I want to be. I think about what's keeping me from reaching that goal. *What is it that I don't want from myself and how can I improve right now?* Depending on my answer, I adjust my affirmation.

I grew up hearing my dad say that rich people weren't good people and to reach that level of success, you had to suffer—it was never something for us to aspire to. If something bad befell someone who was really rich, I'd hear my dad say something like, "Of course, that's what happens when you're rich and greedy," or "That's what happens when you have so much money in your life." Unwittingly, I learned that you had to be miserable and work incessantly to earn every penny because to be otherwise meant that you were a bad person. That mentality stuck with me for a long time, like a negative affirmation. Until one day, when I was already an adult, I went to a seminar based on T. Harv Eker's book *Secrets of the Millionaire Mind*, and I realized something important.

I started studying my life and had to recognize that I'd

achieved a successful, full life. I had to realize that I'd had positive experiences, which were very different from my father's, and there was nothing wrong with that. I didn't have to model my life and my experiences after his; I had to make my own life. That seminar allowed me to believe that I could very well have hundreds of millions of dollars in the bank, that I could speak in terms of thousands instead of hundreds of dollars, and that it was okay to want to earn millions without being a bad person. The more I earn, the more possibilities it lends me to help, motivate, and inspire the next person. The act of aspiring to be well-off economically doesn't mean I have to give up being a humble person with my same values and principles. Moreover, if you're struggling, you can't help others because you're too busy trying to help yourself. The more I have, the more I can serve others.

This experience helped me evolve and refocus my mind, my goals, and my affirmations as I felt the change in me. Finally, I realized that this belief that I could be either rich or happy but not both was not my belief, but my father's. It wasn't true for me. I realized you could be both, and that wanting to make a good salary doesn't make a person unhappy or evil. All of that helped me learn how beliefs and goals have to be as individual as each person's own journey. And that led me to my next affirmation, the one I'm repeating to myself as I write this book: "I am a man who is grateful, healthy, happy, secure, successful, and a billionaire."

I chose **grateful** because so often we are focused on the things we want instead of being thankful for what we have at this moment. I want to affirm my gratefulness for every experience, every second, every opportunity, and every breath.

I say **healthy** because I had some recent troubles with my knee and I want to be healthy enough in my life to continue transforming millions of lives around the world. Moreover, I want my body to be in a perfect state of health and harmony with the infinite universe created by God.

I included the word **happy** because it's an emotion I value greatly, and I always want it present in my life. I want to smile more, and I always want to see the glass as half full.

I'm always working on my self-esteem and that's why I chose the word **secure**. I want to be sure of my decisions and actions. I want those insecurities I still feel daily to be replaced by bravery and strength so I can make the best decisions.

I chose **successful** because I want to invite more success into my life, to see it as something positive, and to free myself from thinking that after a great rise comes a great fall. It's just not that way. We shouldn't be afraid of success. It's something positive in our lives and we deserve to enjoy it.

As for being a **billionaire**, it's one of my long-term goals. I want to think big, which is why I say billionaire and not millionaire. I want to make billions of dollars so I can help billions of people change their lives from the inside out, all over the world. Sometimes, it's still hard for me to believe it, which is why I added it to my affirmation. And remember, it's important to be specific, which is why I said I am a "man," to remind myself that I'm an adult and no longer a boy. If I want to be a billionaire, I can't very well act like a boy. I must act, feel, and value myself as an adult. My affirmation is completely focused on the result I'm trying to achieve *now*. Maybe even by the time you hold this book in your hands, I'll have had to modify it depending on what has happened in my life since.

What constitutes happiness is different for each one of us. We have to find our own path.

The key to all of this is remembering that what constitutes happiness is different for each one of us. We have to find our own path. We can't let ourselves be ruled by what our family, society, or anyone else thinks. We have to be honest with ourselves and find the road that makes each of us happy. That's why your affirmations have to be yours and yours alone. You can't make affirmations or goals to please others, because when you achieve them, they will not make you happy.

Affirmations really have helped me so much and I think they're fundamental to my personal transformation. They keep me aligned with my goals and focused. They keep me continually looking inside myself, without letting myself fall victim to the past. And they help me to defend and define my vision board, which we'll explore in the next chapter on visualization.

Clearly, this process of affirmation has to lead to action. You have to support your words with the appropriate actions, because it doesn't help you to say "I'm slender" if you go out and pound eight hamburgers. Your actions have to be coherent with your words, your thoughts, and your feelings.

I hope you are slowly realizing how interconnected the 7 steps we're discussing in this book really are. It's essential for you to know it because each plays an important role in your transformation, your health, and your well-being. And that's why affirmations go hand in hand with the next step we're going to explore: visualization. I'm glad you're still with me, accompanying me on this marvelous journey to heal your soul. Don't give up now. You're doing a great service to yourself that's going to help you for the rest of your life!

Essential advice to transform your life

- Make an affirmation to lose your emotional weight and heal your soul.
- Get rid of those negative thoughts and transform them into positive energy.
- When you achieve your affirmation, make a new one according to what you want to better or accomplish next.

Put It into Practice!

MAKE YOUR OWN AFFIRMATION

1. If you've paid attention in the previous pages and have followed the suggestions, you should have the three to five words ready to make your affirmation. Remember to start with "I am" and to keep them in the present tense. Be realistic and align them with your goals, so everything works together to help you reach your dreams. Here are a couple examples to give you a push:
   - *I am a healthy, happy, successful man, patiently reaching my goals.*
   - *I am healthy, happy, and proud to be healing my soul and loving my fellow man.*
2. Once you've decided on your affirmation, write it down on a piece of paper or poster board and decorate it with love, because this sentence is going to help you design the new you. You are defining the new person you want to be.
3. Now put the affirmation somewhere you can easily see it every day: in the bathroom, on the refrigerator door, at the foot of your bed. The idea is to repeat the phrase to yourself thirty-three times a day for thirty-three straight days. To make it a habit, I suggest doing it first thing in the morning or just before falling asleep. But if you prefer to do it in the car or the subway on the way to work or while out for a walk, that's fine, too. Do what makes it easy for you to recite it every day.
4. When you recite the words of your affirmation, say them enthusiastically, with conviction and

faith—and a smile. Sing them out loud. Dream of them. Visualize them. Feel them in the depths of your soul. If you want to internalize them more quickly, say them in front of a mirror, looking straight into your eyes. When you do this, you create a direct connection with that chubby little voice that resides inside you, with your heart and soul. Saying these words while looking into your eyes allows your heart and mind to see that the person who is saying these positive things is smiling and happy. It reaffirms that the future person you aspire to be is full of joy and life.

Bery Palomo

My name is Bery Palomo, I'm thirty-three years old, I am Honduran, and I live in the state of Virginia.

I worked as a medical assistant until I became a mother, and with the arrival of my children, I decided to stay home to enjoy watching them grow and to prepare delicious dishes.

I love to cook my Honduran food. Plantains, fried fish, pupusas, baleadas *were part of my daily meal plan and of course I could not contain myself—not my portions or the exaggerated consumption of flour and fat.*

So I was gaining weight until I got to weigh 200 pounds. I had no energy to play with my kids; I was exhausted all the time.

I realized that there wasn't a way to stop my obesity. One day I was getting dressed and I didn't fit into the huge pants I had been using for the last months. I learned that day that I would have to buy a horrible size 15 and extra-large *blouses.*

One of my best friends was going through the same thing. I was desperate to lose weight so we started dieting separately.

I ate only lettuce; other days I stopped eating, drank juices and teas, but nothing helped me get those ugly rolls of fat out of my body. All diets that I've tried were disappointing. I wasn't losing weight and I was gaining pounds instead.

However, my friend's diet seemed to be perfect. She was losing her extra pounds and she could keep eating her Latin meals! Finally she shared her secret with me, her new lifestyle was . . . Yes You Can!

I immediately started my process and it was true. I could cook and enjoy my Latin meals and lose weight in a healthy way.

Today I have lost sixty pounds. I feel beautiful, healthy, and prosperous. Today I achieved the balance with Yes You Can! essential components: nutrition, emotional health, movement, and success.

Thanks for changing my life, Yes You Can!

SUCCESS STORY

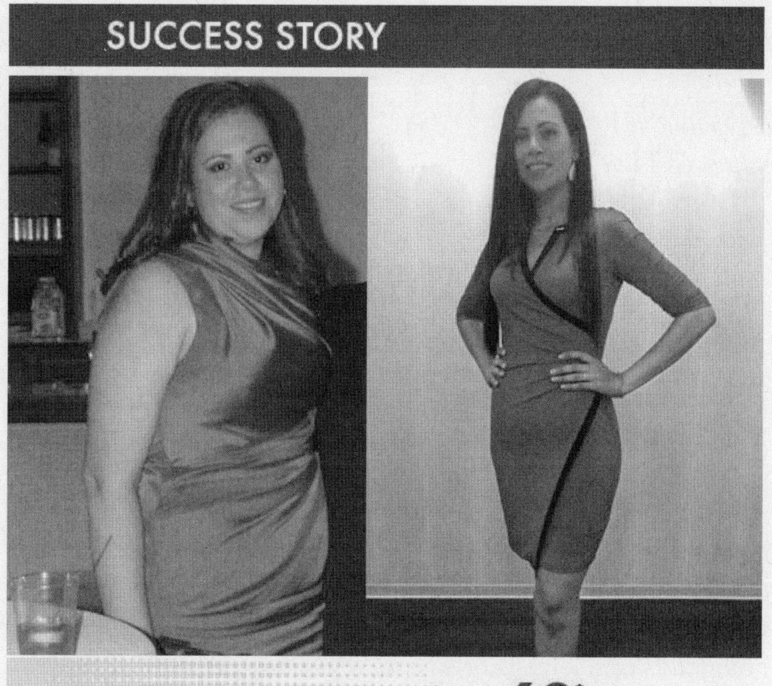

BERY PALOMO **lost 60* lbs**

BERY'S ADVICE: *Perseverance is the key to achieving your goals. Do not give up and know that every day that passes gets you closer to your transformation and that is your engine or motivation. I love to cook and to learn how to do it in a healthy way from the nutrition guide that came with my Food Lover kit, which was a tremendous help.*

There are a few words I'd like to say to you: Yes You Can!

**Results not typical and will vary according to diet, exercise, metabolism, and genetic makeup.*

(EIGHT)

Step 5: Visualize Your Dream Life

THE POWER OF words is magical, and so is the power of the mind, imagination, and visualization. Visualizations are what we imagine we can one day achieve. It starts with the images in our head, which make us dream big. It's what we used to do as children. Didn't we, as kids, all dream about what we would be when we grew up? Some of us wanted to be actors or astronauts or firefighters or scientists or singers. The possibilities were endless.

That's the beauty of childhood. When we're kids, we don't have as many fears. We think everything is possible and that keeps us from limiting ourselves. This is what I want for you. I want you to break those restrictions adulthood forces on us in order to allow yourself to dream big. Let your imagination run wild.

Imagination is the ability to create an idea, a mental image, or a feeling. Visualization uses our imagination to create a clear representation of something we want to come true. It helps us transform our dreams into reality.

Imagine what a day would be like for a healthy person who doesn't have the compulsion to eat, who doesn't crave a bite when toxic emotions wash over her. Picture that person in your head. Now replace that person's face with your own and *visualize* the same thing. Can you see yourself?

- Visualize yourself happy, free, focused on your goals, achieving your dreams.

- Visualize yourself doing what you most want to do.
- Visualize yourself without any fear.
- Visualize yourself a winner.
- Visualize yourself successful and financially secure.
- Visualize yourself at the moment you've achieved your goals for the year.

How does that make your feel? Write it down. I want you to remember this sensation of joy, freedom, satisfaction, limitlessness, because that's what you should feel during your visualizations.

THE LAW OF ATTRACTION AND VISUALIZATION GO HAND IN HAND

We have the power to create and attract exactly what we think, feel, imagine, say, write, and visualize. For example, many Olympic athletes practice not only on the field but in their minds, imagining perfect execution in their day-to-day training as much as in their ultimate triumph. They close their eyes and visualize the moment to the point where they can feel the gold medal being draped around their necks, listening to the crowd's thunderous applause. They visualize the reality they desire and they connect it to their goals, so they can feel it at their fingertips, more attainable than ever.

All of this is directly related to the Law of Attraction, which states that all our beliefs and thoughts influence what we attract in our lives. If you spend the day thinking about the negative, all of the things you don't have, all the bad things in your life, how sad you are, and what frustrates you, you are only attracting more negativity, frustration, and sadness into your life. But you can change this! If instead of thinking of all the negativity in your day-to-day life you start to think about all the positive things, you will attract more and more positive moments, things, and people.

I can guess what you're thinking: "Oh, Alejandro, some

days everything just goes wrong for me. How can I focus on the positive when it's all negative?" I'm sure that something good happens to you in the course of a day. However, so often we're closed to the good things because we're blinded by the negative. But okay, for the sake of argument, let's say you've had one of those days where nothing is going your way. If you honestly can't think of anything good that happened to you on a given day, I want you, just before you fall asleep, to set aside a few minutes to express gratitude (something we should do every day, whether it was a good or a bad day). Thank God and the Universe for being alive, for being healthy, for the fact that your eyes function and you can see, for having feet and legs that allow you to walk, for the bed you're lying in, for everything that has been given to you. For your dog. For your kids. For being in this country. For your job. For everything you *do* have.

> *The stones you feel life has put in your way are actually ones you put there yourself.*

When you do this, you're filling yourself with positive energy. And you know what? That's something good you can give thanks for! It's all in your hands. The stones you feel life has put in your way are actually ones you put there yourself. It all starts with you. Once you start to untangle your feelings and see the positive things in your life, you'll witness how little by little they start multiplying themselves. And that will attract more positive moments in your life.

Thinking positive and being grateful are two key tools that will help you find your happiness. They go hand in hand with affirmations and visualizations, which will help you choose the right path in life: the positive path over the negative. C'mon, you can do this! You deserve it!

VISUALIZE YOUR BEST SELF

You can't imagine how important visualization was to me when I was losing weight. I'd close my eyes and could see, hear, and feel myself at the beach, swimming without a shirt on. I'd cut out the svelte bodies I so admired and paste them on poster boards next to inspirational quotes all over my house. I did everything I could to picture myself having met my goal, wearing a size 30 waist, my body lean, and a smile on my face.

Visualize yourself the way you want to be. How do you visualize your slender self? What would you do first? What would it feel like to get out of bed? What would you wear? Where would you go? What would you say? How would you act? Our brain works by creating images. We respond daily to different memories that flash into our mind or that we carry around in our subconscious. To modify our reaction to those memories, we need to introduce new images to our mind. Think about how children learn to speak and write. Teachers always use images. For example, if we're trying to teach a child the word "sun," we show her a picture of a sun over and over so she can associate that sound, that syllable, with the image. Without the image, the child could never identify the sun. That's how important images are in our lives.

YOUR VISION BOARD

One of the keys to visualization is creating your vision board. This is the place where we can express the things we desire in life in full-color images. It's basically your visualization expressed on a poster board. The idea is to place images on it that represent your goals. It's a visual representation of how we want our new year to look, of all the things we want to achieve. It's an excellent way to put the Law of Attraction to work.

When you set out to create your vision board, be sure to

be clear and specific, just as you were with your goals and affirmations. Each detail you use on your vision board is important. I have a friend who put what she thought was the man of her dreams on her vision board. He had all the characteristics she was looking for, down to the color of his hair, eyes, and how he dressed. At least, that's what she thought. One fine day, she met a man who took her breath away. He was exactly as she had described him on her vision board. She couldn't be happier.

Nevertheless, as she got to know him, problems started to arise. The guy was an alcoholic. Her dream was demolished in a single blow. That definitely wasn't something she wanted in a relationship and she decided to end it. She was sad and decided to revise her vision board. When she looked closely at it, she realized the person she had cut out had a drink in his hand. She was stupefied! That's why we have to be so careful with the images we put on our vision board: The universe will send us *exactly* what we ask for.

At the same time, you have to be realistic. You can't ask for the impossible. And there's another detail, which isn't a minor one. You have to use color images, not black and white. One year, a friend decided to use black and white images for her vision board. It looked beautiful. But nothing she put on her vision board came to pass that year. What she didn't know is that the mind doesn't process black and white images the same way it does color ones. The mind tends to make them disappear, to the point that some neurolinguistic programming experts will even tell you to picture someone who treats you badly in black and white, and they will disappear from your mind. Besides, things in color are more vivid and feel more real. At the end of the day, we experience life in color, and that's how we should see our desires as projected on our vision boards.

Following these key suggestions, you can go about building your vision board however you like. You can trace pictures, cut out photos from magazines, write inspirational phrases, or draw or paint your own images. I like using pictures I find in magazines or on Google. Sometimes, I Photoshop my face into a scene, from a happy family to an interview with Oprah. I place the Yes You Can! logo on countries around the world that I know we will one day reach. I design the cover of books I'm working on and write "No. 1 *New York Times* Bestseller" across the front. All that and much more.

The goal is to cover every aspect of your life, from professional to personal. In one of the boards I made when I was losing weight, I put a picture of a slender person. He wasn't a model, just someone who was thinner than I was at the time. When I reached that weight, I edited my board to show my next goal, a man with slightly more defined muscles. And then I edited it again to show a model with larger muscles. And then with cut abs. It evolved over time according to my path. It's a way to make yourself believe that image is possible in your own life.

Just as with your goals and affirmations, you have to update your vision board depending on what occurs in your life. I like doing mine on my birthday. Another good time to do it is at the start of a new year. When you do it is totally up to you. But don't stop yourself from revising it during the course of the year as things change in your life. For example, if you're in a relationship and it suddenly comes to an end, it's advisable to edit this part of your treasure map toward a new goal. It's happened to me, and when it did, I took down photos of us on trips I visualized us taking and replaced them with images that reflected my new circumstance, whether that was to find someone else or work on myself for a while. Life is constant change, and our goals, affirmations, and visualizations should reflect that. In my case, I still had many challenges to face, but without them, I wouldn't be the person I am today.

> *Life is constant change, and our goals, affirmations, and visualizations should reflect that.*

FROM IMAGINATION TO REALITY

When I was a boy living in a small town, I liked to look up at the night sky and wonder what we looked like from another world. I was a curious child and I wanted to have new experiences in other parts of the world. I also dreamed of being an actor and loved imagining myself one day on the cover of *People en Español*. It didn't seem impossible. It felt like a distant goal, but still when it came to mind, I would laugh and think to myself, *Wow, can you imagine?*

By the end of the year 2000, I had reached my goal of becoming a professional actor and I was approaching another: to live abroad. The network I acted on decided to move me to Miami, so I could act in the *telenovelas* that are filmed there. The little boy from Maturín with big dreams never could have imagined that in a few years, he'd be moving to this place that would become his new home.

For me, moving from Maturín to Caracas was a dream come true. I finally had access to more information and used it to reach my goals. But landing in Miami was a whole other level. All of a sudden, I was in a place filled with competition, where the ripped and svelte bodies all around me were the best I'd ever seen in my life. As I found my way, the same thing happened to me that happens to a lot of us when we arrive in a new country: I gained a little weight. It wasn't much, but I felt so swollen. For someone who had been obese, it was a red flag. I had no idea what was happening to me. I hadn't changed my eating habits, but the ingredients were different, and they were clearly affecting my body. When I called my trainer in Caracas, he told me my body was likely retaining water and that I should try to buy all organic products. Great idea, sure. But I wasn't making the kind of money that allowed me to go crazy at the supermarket. I hadn't moved because of a big paycheck but for the chance to gain acting experience and to live in the United States.

I spent four uneasy, bloated months in Miami, worried about regaining weight. I was terrified at the prospect of having to wear size 38 pants and XL shirts again. I wasn't sure what to do. Thinking that the diet that had worked so well for me in Venezuela was no longer effective, I started looking for other alternatives. I went through a phase where I tried every single diet in Miami, from the South Beach Diet to Jenny Craig, even Weight Watchers. Nothing seemed to work. I never understood how someone could live his or her whole life eating prepackaged food. After the third frozen dinner, I threw in the towel. Those fake brownies tasted horrible and I never fully got the hang of the Weight Watchers points. It was all so complicated. I needed something easier that I could rely on in the hustle and bustle of my daily life. I decided to return to my diet from Venezuela, following it to the letter, eating super clean, without cheating even once, not just for my health but for my career. And I finally found a balance.

Over the next three years I lived in Miami, and not only did I work on different *telenovelas* but I also finished my law degree. Although I had left school and acting was going so well for me, my dad was still unhappy with the situation. He said he'd invested too much for me just to leave school half-finished. He said it so often that one day I blurted out, "Don't worry, Dad, I'll get you that diploma one day." I reenrolled in college and finished my degree online. And in 2003, I got my law degree. I skipped graduation because it was something I'd done for my father, not for myself. But I was able to give him that much. I handed him my diploma and he happily hung it in his office, and I kept going down my own path.

At the beginning of 2004, I was chosen to be in a new *tele-*

novela, but the filming would be in Dallas. And with that came another change in my life that caused me stress, no thanks to the emotional weight I was still dealing with. Since I'd gained weight when I first moved to Miami, I lived in fear of gaining weight once I moved to Dallas. I was terrified that anything new I ate would make me put on pounds. But that didn't stop me. Sometimes I cheated on my diet and that drove me crazy. I felt such a terrible guilt that I never even enjoyed the cheat food. For example, I'd eat an ice cream and by the time I tossed the cup in the trash, I'd start to feel regret. *Why did I eat that? Now I'm screwed. Look at my cellulite . . .* My mind was my worst enemy. I'd start over the next week, stricter than ever, doing more cardio than usual, being mindful of every bite of food I put in my mouth. But by Sunday, I was off track again, gorging on food and immediately regretting it. It was a vicious cycle.

Although my mind and emotions tormented me for each lapse, I was actually in great shape. I was playing the role of a boxer in Dallas and dove head first into finding out about that lifestyle. I started basing my diet on what a boxer eats and I was stronger and leaner than I'd ever been. As I should be, since that was my job.

Meanwhile, the move to Dallas revealed to me that I really couldn't speak English very well. In Miami, you speak so much Spanish that you barely need to speak English. The little I knew made me feel like a local. But the second I stepped foot in Texas, reality hit and a new goal was born: to learn English.

Thanks to a colleague in Dallas, I decided that after the *telenovela* ended, I would move to Los Angeles. She told me that in LA, not only could I improve my English but I'd also have a chance at auditioning for English-speaking roles. *Wow, what an opportunity! I'd be in Hollywood!* I thought to myself, *If Antonio Banderas could do it, why not me?* When the *telenovela* wrapped, I packed my bags and headed toward my new goal.

I studied English for a year, and when I felt more comfortable with it, I started auditioning in English. Out of thirty or forty auditions, I only got one call back. All those "nos" seemed to outweigh the one "yes." But that didn't stop me. In time, thanks to effort, passion, and perseverance, I started landing little roles here and there, until one day I was selected to play a role on an HBO series titled *Twelve Miles of Bad Road*, which would be filmed in Texas, and where I would be acting alongside American actors such as the great Lily Tomlin. I jumped at the chance. Not only would I get to play alongside a great cast, it came with another huge plus: the salary. Compared to what I was making doing *telenovelas,* I felt like Bill Gates—something that would eventually work against me.

Luckily I wasn't having any issues with my diet at that point. I had all the tools to help me create a personalized diet. Without realizing it, I was creating a new diet that was working for me and was based on everything I'd learned. It was the beginning of what a few years later would become Yes You Can!

With the money I made on this new acting job, I took out a loan to buy a house in Los Angeles and the car of my dreams. It didn't occur to me to save anything. I had no concept of what a budget was. I figured money was made to be spent. I was enjoying my success, yet I still had this belief that having money was bad. Because of this belief and not having the right information, I spent every dollar I made. I had no idea of the headache that was on the horizon.

In 2008, the series we were filming in Texas was cancelled. Not only was I out of a job, but the U.S. economic crisis took hold and my house in Los Angeles lost 60 percent of its value. In the blink of an eye, I found myself back in Los Angeles without a job, without any auditions lined up, paying a huge mortgage, and with no idea what to do next.

On top of everything, I felt lonely in Los Angeles. It's an expansive city where the neighborhoods are miles apart and you can end up feeling very isolated. I had a close friend who was also an actress, but she lived on the opposite side of town. No matter how much we wanted to hang out, we couldn't justify the hours of traffic and gas it would take to see each other on an average weeknight.

Nevertheless, I never ran back to food for comfort. Food had stopped being a problem. I think everything I had learned the years before helped me reach a place of maturity and clarity. I finally had all the tools at my disposal and was starting to use them in my favor—at least with food.

But in my other new circumstances, I felt truly lost and desperate. Not only was I living in a house worth half the amount I was paying, but my credit cards were all maxed out and I had only $240 in my checking account. I kept going to auditions but never got any callbacks. I needed to land a big role to get out of this mess, since it was the only thing I'd learned to do to make a living. And I definitely didn't want to ask my dad for help.

He had always done well in his business, but the Venezuelan economy was also going from bad to worse. Everyone was affected, including my dad. Plus after all the times he warned me about going into acting, I was too embarrassed to ask him for help. I kept it to myself for a long time. I only mentioned how frustrated I was when I was passed up for a role. The only thing my father would say was, "Forget all that. You can come work here." He still didn't understand my desire to be an actor and I wasn't ready to tell him I had found myself in a huge, unexpected financial hole with no idea how to get out.

I consulted an attorney who said that given my current situation and mounting debt, my best option was to declare bankruptcy. Bankruptcy! Yes, it was the only way out. Filled with doubts, fears, frustration, and sadness, I signed the mountains of paperwork and when the lawyer handed me his bill, I nearly fainted. Twelve thousand dollars! What do you mean, twelve thousand dollars? With two hundred bucks in the bank and my credit shot because of the bankruptcy, where was I going to get that kind of money? I was tormented by anxiety and felt myself slipping into total desperation.

I still didn't look for refuge in food, but that stress and that anxiety caused me so much emotional weight that my mind screamed out for some kind of escape. That's how I got into smoking and soon cigarettes became my best friends. My favorite saying became, "God, I'm so stressed! I need a cigarette!" I was a walking chimney. I had found a new way to cover up what I was feeling, but I didn't realize it until much later, when I finally quit. The little money I had I spent on cigarettes and food at 99-cent stores.

So now I was still without a job, without any money, bankrupt, and I had a twelve-thousand-dollar debt! I needed to do something and fast. So I got on Craigslist and came across a job as a clown for kids' birthday parties. Perfect! Finally, a job I was qualified to do as an actor. I called about the job and got it. I breathed a sign of relief, went out to buy the cheapest clown outfit and makeup I could find, and got to work. So every weekend, I painted my face white, packed my clown gear into a bag, and drove off to that week's jobs. It turned out to be easier than I had imagined. Sure, it was a huge blow to my self-esteem to try to make people laugh while I was going through one of the worst periods of my adult life, filled with doubt and feeling like my dreams had come crashing down. But it was just what I had to do to survive.

During the week, I'd gotten a job at the fast food chicken chain El Pollo Loco. I started out washing the raw chicken and soon worked my way up to cashier. The job was another huge challenge. I had to look my ego square in the face. I wasn't famous at the time but well known enough that every now and then, someone would come to the front of the line and say, "Wait, I know you. You're the guy from the *telenovela*!" God, at those moments, I just wanted the earth to swallow me up. I wanted to disappear. Dressed in my El Pollo Loco uniform, with the smell of fried chicken coming out of my pores, I had no choice but to suck up my disappointment, sadness, and humiliation and say with a smile, "Yup, that's me. So what can I get for you?"

I had two choices: cry and feel sorry for myself or lift my head and keep moving forward. I decided to keep fighting. I worked seven days a week, five at El Pollo Loco and the weekends as a clown. I'd arrived in Hollywood as an actor trying to find my way. Incredible opportunities opened their doors to me and everything looked like it was going according to plan. Then, in the blink of an eye, I went from a film set to manning the register at El Pollo Loco. Today, I realize it was the best thing that could have happened to me because I learned valuable lessons that will last a lifetime. But at the moment it sure didn't feel that way.

I came home smelling like chicken. I worked constantly, but don't think I gave up on acting. If I was called in for an audition, I changed in the El Pollo Loco bathroom, ran to my car, tossed my uniform in the back, and took off to the audition, thinking, *God, don't let these people say, "Uh, why do you smell like refried beans?"* I was doing everything in my power to get out of this hole. But there were days when I wanted to run away and disappear. Yet even though I was filled with doubts, giving up was not an option.

When I declared bankruptcy, I had to turn in my car and move out of my house. I spent the first two months at a friend's house, and she was like an angel who opened her doors to me when I needed it most. I remember that one of my first days there, I stepped out onto her balcony and my eyes filled with tears that flowed like a torrent. I was so hopeless, so beaten, so lost. I thought, *What do I do now? Where do I start?* There were nights I lay down to sleep and thought I was in a horror movie. I asked myself, *What did I do to deserve this? Why is this happening to me? What went wrong? Whom did I hurt? Where is this karma coming from?*

In those moments, we never understand why we're going

through all that. Everything feels dark and we can't even see the light at the end of the tunnel. I was about to turn twenty-seven and I had nothing in the world but my dog, Azul. And even that brought it's own challenges. I had a pair of reading glasses someone had given me that cost $700. I never took them off for anything. One night, I fell asleep with them while reading *The Alchemist* (looking for signs of hope) in bed with my dog. At midnight, I woke up, put them on the nightstand, and fell back asleep. I never imagined my pup would think my glasses were her new chew toy. The next morning when I opened my eyes and felt around for my glasses, I found what was left of them. They were chewed to bits. God, I was so angry! I wanted to kill Azul! But how could I even think that of my pup, my beautiful Azul, whom I loved so much and was the only thing I had left in this world that gave me unconditional love. So now, on top of everything else, I couldn't even see well and was prone to headaches from squinting all day.

Those are the moments when we have to look for a ray of light, hold on to God, and have faith that He has a plan for us. Believe me, I know it's not easy. The only thing I kept wondering was why this had happened to me. There were moments I thought, *Maybe it's better if I just get hit by a bus and get this over with.* I didn't realize that by filling myself with negative thoughts, I was attracting more negativity into my life. But I didn't know what else to do.

Nevertheless, that's exactly the moment when we have to change our attitude and transform those incessant questions that take over our thoughts into something positive. Of course, we're not immediately going to see it through rose-colored glasses. But we can replace at least one negative thought with one positive thought. Yes, I was going through one of the hardest phases of my life, but I was lucky enough to find gainful employment. And I was fortunate to have a great friend who took me in when I had no one else. Within two months, I was able to rent myself a little studio I could call my own.

Was I living my dream? No. But I was taking baby steps back toward my path. I bought myself a mattress and a chair at IKEA. Aside from my computer, those were the only two things I had in my studio. That and faith. Sticking to God and the values my parents had taught me since I was a boy, I kept doing honest work, praying, going to church in search of peace. At night I'd go to sleep while praying, asking for the strength to keep moving forward in God's path. After one particularly hard, painful day, when I'd asked God for a sign and the guidance and strength to keep going, I got a phone call that seemed heaven-sent.

"Chabán," said the producer of the *telenovela* I'd worked on in Dallas. "I'm calling you because I'm shooting a new *telenovela* and want to know if I can count on you for one of the lead roles. I think it'd be perfect for you and I want it to be you."

"Absolutely, I'm in," I said. Thank God, the lease I'd signed was month to month.

"But I haven't even told you what it pays," he replied.

"Doesn't matter. All I'm asking is that you fly me there. I need to get out of here. I need something to give me hope again."

Two weeks later, I was in Miami, signing the contract. In just two weeks, my life had turned around. I was starting a new phase of my life that would allow me to achieve things that just two weeks earlier seemed unimaginable. With that new job, not only was I able to pay off the lawyer, but another visualization I'd made as a boy was about to come true. When *Eva Luna* aired and we went on a press junket to promote it, it was a huge success. Coverage was everywhere. And out of the blue, I got a call one day from *People en Español*: They'd chosen *me* as one of their 50 Most Beautiful People! This was really happening! The chubby little kid was being called one of the 50 Most Beautiful! It seemed like a dream. When I got my hands on a copy of the magazine and read what it said about me, I was awestruck. It said I was the new hunk at Univision and that the audience was in love. Me? A hunk? I'd never imagined that the sad, chubby little boy who was constantly ridiculed could one day be considered a heart throb. But there it was, in black and white; everything I'd been working for was materializing before my very eyes. No one knew what it had taken for me to get there. As the saying goes, "You can never judge a man until you've walked a mile in his moccasins."

GET READY TO ENJOY THE FRUITS OF YOUR VISUALIZATIONS

The things you visualize can become reality when you least expect it. When you turn your problems over to God, work hard, and hold on to your faith, the blessings come flooding into your life. This isn't a theory I learned in a book. I'm telling you this because I've lived it. Our thoughts, the Law of Attraction, and the power of God are all incredible forces. And they are available to all of us. All we have to do is have faith, believe in God, and take action to apply this faith to our lives.

I believe devoutly in all of this, just as I do in the vision board, because I've been a witness to it: If God has deemed me worthy of having something, it has come true. Sometimes it takes longer than you think, but if it's what God and the Universe wants for us, it all comes in time. I visualized being in *People en Español* and now I had the magazine to prove it had come true. I visualized the car of my dreams, and now it's parked outside my house. I visualized being on the cover of *Men's Health* and that dream came true, too. I visualized my dream apartment and now I live in it. I'd even visualized something else years earlier—something I'd completely forgotten about—and it was my best friend who reminded me that it came true as well.

When I was offered to be a host on *Despierta América*, I was honored. But I wasn't sure if I could meet the time demands and get up at 3:30 a.m. every day. I was going back and forth on it; I wasn't sure what to do. So I called my best friend to talk it over and she immediately reminded me of something.

"Wait just a minute. Don't you remember the vision board we made when you arrived in Miami in 2000?"

"No, I don't," I said.

"Well, I'm going to send you the picture. I have it here. Wait until you see it."

When she emailed me the picture, I nearly fainted. I'd put a picture of the hosts of *Despierta América* on my vision board. *Wow,* I thought, *this can't be!* I didn't need to think about it anymore. I accepted the offer and it has been one of the best decisions I've ever made. I can reach a wider audience to help more people, I can put some joy into people's mornings, and I feel I am fulfilling my purpose in life. Not to mention that I get to work with some truly exceptional people for whom I'm grateful every morning.

That's what ultimately made me believe that our future truly lies in our hands, in our minds, and in our hearts. It all depends on our words, our thoughts, and our imagination. The more emphasis we put on the good and positive things in our lives, the more we focus on our goals, affirmations, and visualizations, the closer we get to accomplishing them. Each of these steps is essential. But there's one thing that's crystal clear: Without action, there are no results. If you sit on your couch reciting your affirmations and looking at your vision board without actually going out and looking for the path that will lead you to your goals, you won't accomplish anything. Your goals aren't going to come knocking on your door. Your dreams aren't magically going to come sailing in through a window. Now that your mind and heart are focused on your purpose in life, it's time to take action. Don't be afraid. It's an emotional ride, and nothing can replace the joy and satisfaction of reaching your goals. I know you can do it!

Put It into Practice!

HOW TO MAKE A VISION BOARD

Ingredients

- Your list of goals
- Magazines to cut out pictures (You can also search the Internet for pictures, print them, and cut them out.)
- Scissors
- Scotch tape or white glue
- Colored markers
- Anything you might want to help decorate your vision board

Directions

1. Look for images in magazines or on the Internet that represent your goals and print them or cut them out.
2. Once you've cut them all out, start taping or pasting them onto the board. It doesn't matter where you place them. Picture this as a collage made up of your dreams.
3. If you want to be more specific, use your markers to write things next to the images. It could be words, phrases, or pictures. It could be your name. Whatever will help you create the most detailed and clear images of your goals.
4. Repeat the previous steps for all the pictures that represent your goals. If you want, write positive phrases in the white spaces, things like "love," or "prosperity," or "health." You can decorate it any way you like. The goal is for the final product to make you smile and fill you with joy

and inspiration. Those are the images you've chosen to represent you. Let yourself think big. Don't limit yourself! Let your imagination guide you toward your dreams.

5. Once it's ready, put your vision board somewhere visible, perhaps your bedroom or your office. You can even take a picture of it and make it into your screensaver. Every time you see it, try to connect with the images. Feel them. I want it to inspire joy and hope so you can achieve everything your heart desires. You deserve it!

Sofía Ballester

My name is Sofía Ballester. I'm eighteen years old and I'm Puerto Rican. A year ago, I weighed 264 pounds and knew what it was like to be bullied at school. I bit my lip in shame as people used me as the butt of their jokes, and told me I walked like an elephant. Amid so much loneliness and sadness I just wanted to find a few instances of joy and I'd find it in food. I'd buy pastries and fried food, and come home to eat it all, alone with plates full of roast pork, rice and beans, yucca, and plenty of ice cream.

As my prom neared, I weighed 264 pounds and was ashamed to put on my prom dress. Plus, because of how overweight I was, no one wanted to go with me. In February of that year, I discovered Yes You Can! when Alejandro Chabán gave a speech in Puerto Rico. His words helped me make the decision that "Yes, I could, too." I started the plan and learned tools that would help me reach my goal of losing weight.

I saw results from the very first week. I started losing weight by eating healthy food that I enjoyed.

I went to prom after all and left everyone with mouths agape. The new Sofía had lost seventy-five pounds and dropped from a size XXL to a medium. Thank you, Alejandro Chabán, for being the prince who saved my life and helped me become a secure young woman. I feel I can continue on this future journey of achieving my goals. Today, I can say with pride, Yes You Can!

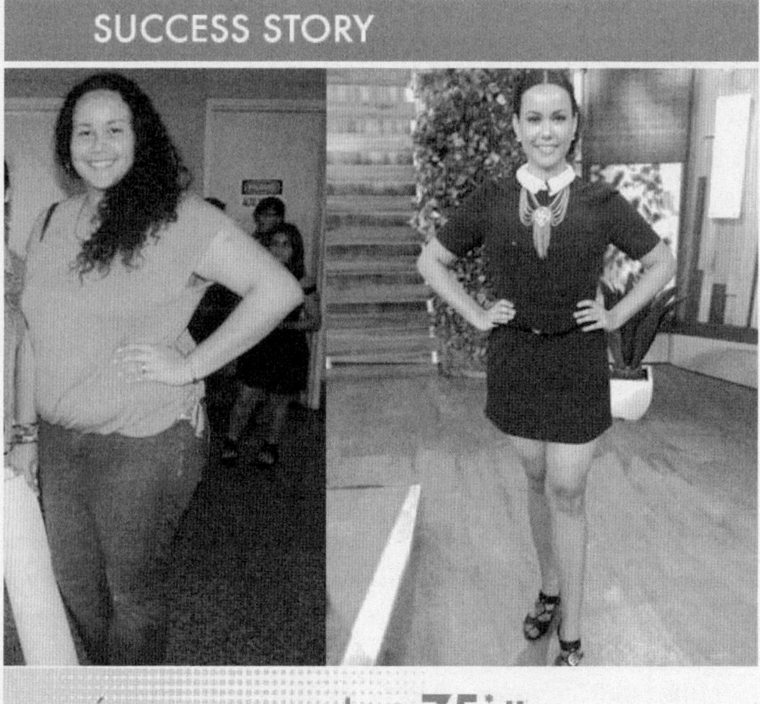

SOFÍA'S ADVICE: *What helped me was taking my protein shakes with me to school, no matter what my classmates said. Sometimes, I had to stay up late studying and that fat-free, sugar-free shake helped me quell my hunger pangs while I finished, and it helped me go to bed full.*

**Results not typical and will vary according to diet, exercise, metabolism, and genetic makeup.*

(NINE)

Step 6: Take Action and Create Lasting Habits

SO FAR, YOU'VE committed to yourself, identified your emotional weight, defined and written down your goals, and you've used them to create your affirmations and vision board. Congrats! Now, it's time to take action. Intent plus action equals transformation. Everything you want also wants you—but you have to take action to obtain it. Otherwise, it will only ever be an illusion.

> *Everything you want also wants you—but you have to take action to obtain it.*

Every morning, I do my breathing exercises and I repeat my affirmations out loud. And every night, before I go to bed, I look at my vision board to focus my mind on the images of what I want most in my life. Plus, I write down ten things I'm grateful for. But the only way these magical words and images can become reality is through actions. Every time you set new goals, start working toward them immediately. Otherwise you'll lose the passion and those goals will simply become a memory.

In that block of time between when I say my affirmations in the morning and when I look at my vision board at night, I set out to put my plan into action, and to keep taking the steps I need to reach my destination. Where there's a will, there's a way. Don't let fear paralyze you. The moment you're ready to spring into action, there will be a thousand reasons cropping up to try to sabotage you. "It's too hard. It's too rough. It's dangerous. It's boring. It's tedious. It's too expensive. I don't like it." Let it fall on deaf ears and *just do* the things that will lead you toward success. The moment you take action, that fear evaporates.

You can talk to death all the things you *could* do or *want to* do. But until you begin, these are only words. When you create a plan without action, these goals, affirmations, and visualizations become only wishes.

The most successful people in life are the ones who act courageously, make decisions, and are willing to take risks.

The most successful people in life are the ones who act courageously, make decisions, and are willing to take risks. I know that sometimes it's easier said than done because our fears, beliefs, and excuses are stronger than our desire to act. That's why I've come up with a motto that has always helped me when I'm facing some kind of fear, and I hope it can help you: "Fear is like a snake that we'll never be able to kill, eliminate, destroy, or even shrink. We can only tame it." How? By taking action.

If you want to reach your goals, if you want to transform your affirmations and visualizations into reality, then you need to *act*. Action is the bridge between desire and reality. There's no way around that bridge. Our only options are to stay on one side of that bridge with our desires unfulfilled, or cross it toward our passion, toward that need that God has placed in our hearts. You need massive and determined action. Don't give up. Keep trying and taking action until you reach your objective. When your child is learning to walk, and she falls the first time, what do you tell her? "Try again!" She tries again, falls again. What do you say now? "Try again!" You'd never say, "Ah, well, you tried a couple times. Maybe it's better if you don't walk." You have to get over the fear that keeps you from moving and just start, nothing more, nothing less. Of course, the journey won't always be easy. You'll probably run up against things you won't like, unexpected surprises, distractions, obstacles, people, and situations that slow you down. You may deviate from your path at times, but you have to keep pushing forward until you cross to the other side of the bridge.

Beware: The closer you get to your goals, to reaching the other side of the bridge, to achieving success, the more people will appear to try to distract you and put obstacles in your way. This is when you have to stay the most focused. This is the moment when life tests you—the moment of truth. This is when you have to be your strongest, more powerful than all the obstacles in your path. It's as if the universe is testing your resolve to see if you truly are ready to receive this prize you want and deserve.

YOUR DECISIONS PLAY A VITAL ROLE IN YOUR ACTIONS

There is a famous song called "Decisiones" by singer Rubén Blades. Loosely translated, the chorus is: *Decisions every day / Someone loses, someone wins / Ave Maria!* Every person in the song makes a decision that drastically affects his or her life. And it's like that for all of us, too. We have the power in our hands to make decisions that affect our future. That's why it's so important to pay attention and learn to make better choices in our lives. The smaller the details, the more they affect us.

Every decision you make affects the next one.

Every decision you make affects the next one. For example, when someone serves us a huge plate of creamy coconut rice, we have to decide whether we're going to partake. We ask ourselves, "Should I eat it or not?" Regardless of whether we're heavy or skinny, we all ask ourselves this question. It's a matter of whether our decision falls in line with our goals. In our case, if we want to be healthy, if we want to untether our emotions from food, and someone offers us something decadent and fattening, the best decision is to say no. It may be tough, but later we're going to feel good about ourselves. And that satisfied feeling is what's going to help us to keep moving forward.

Don't let yourself be manipulated by others. Maybe it's your grandma who's offering you dessert and when you say no, she lays in with the guilt. "But I made it just for you because I know it's your favorite!" "I cooked it with so much love. Take just a little bite, won't you?" If you're not firm in your decision, the one you know is best for you, these phrases we know too well could derail you from your goal. You might find yourself eating that dessert just to make someone else happy, an action that goes against the new, good habits you're trying to establish.

Moreover, if you give up and eat the dessert, you're not only derailing your diet and your goal of losing weight, but you're also telling your brain that your word is no good and you haven't really made a commitment to yourself. You're telling your brain, "I'm a liar. Don't pay attention when I have something to say because I don't make good on my promises." You have to be true to your word and truly respect your commitment to yourself. Otherwise, your mind won't believe what you say. If you say, "I'm starting my diet today," and you quit two weeks later, or "I'm going to quit smoking," and have a cigarette in hand three weeks after, or "I'm taking computer classes starting today," but you get bored and give up, you're only conditioning your mind to not believe in your own resolutions. If you repeat this habit over and over, your mind will become accustomed to you not keeping your word. The next time you say, "Today, I'm going to start exercising," your mind will say subtly, "I'll believe it when I see it." It's a domino effect that only sets you back.

If you set out a plate of asparagus and a slice of cake and ask me which one I want, I'm going to say cake. Of course I'm going to *want* cake. But which one is going to ensure that I fit into my size 32 pants next month? The asparagus. That moment—that decision—is the key. You have to replace the urge at that very moment with your goal's intention. Think about whether your decision will add or subtract on your journey: Is that slice of pizza going to help me or hinder me in my goal? It may not be what you *want* to do but what you *have* to do that should guide your decision.

> *To reach your goals and achieve your dreams, there are things you* have *to do whether you want to or not.*

Let's be clear: Not everything we do will be for the pure desire of doing it. To reach your goals and achieve your dreams, there are things you *have* to do whether you want to or not. To lose weight, like it or not, you have to eat five times a day, include protein in your diet, stay in motion, measure your portions, burn more calories than you consume, drink plenty of water, and eliminate sugar. Nothing frustrates me more than spending fifteen minutes talking with someone who says they're dying to lose weight only to end the conversation with them telling me, "Oh, I can't live without my beer, cheese, or bacon." That person isn't ready to lose weight. She won't make the decisions necessary to reach her goals because she hasn't taken the first step: making a commitment to herself.

See how important each of the 7 steps is and how they relate to each other? If you don't make a commitment to yourself, when it comes time to make decisions, you won't take the actions required to change your bad habits and create lasting good ones. Everything goes hand in hand. You can't take one step without the others being aligned. How can you possibly let a beer or cheese or bacon stand between you and your goal of losing those extra pounds? How often have you had beer or chocolate in your life? You mean to tell me you can't live without these things for some time in order to reach your goal of losing weight?

If you really want something and you've already committed to yourself, established clear goals, made affirmations, and are using visualization, it's time to ask yourself, "What am I physically doing toward that goal?" What actions am I taking to achieve that desire? Is your answer really nothing? Really? You're doing nothing to reach that goal? Then you can forget it because you're never going to accomplish it that way.

Action always has to go hand in hand with your goals, and those are related to the decisions you make every day. We make choices every minute and we have to make sure they're the choices that lead us down the right path. You want to lose weight? Good. So when someone offers you dessert, you have to make the decision and say no. If you eat the dessert, you're furthering yourself from your goal. I have friends who complain about being unemployed but they don't go out to find a job. They don't sit down to make calls or search the Internet for prospects. Their goal is to find a job but their actions don't reflect that goal. If you really need employment, then go out and find it! You think I wanted to work as a clown or at El Pollo Loco? Of course not. But I had fallen off my track and I had to do whatever it took to get back on the route that would take me to my goals.

I want to be extra clear here: Reaching your goals is no easy task. It requires a lot of effort, perseverance, and a huge dose of patience, since many of these goals won't be realized right away. It could take weeks or months, even years. But that doesn't mean you should give up.

Too often we make decisions based on what we want at that very moment instead of taking into account what we need to do to meet our long-term goals. That's why it's important to establish clear goals. Otherwise we make decisions without thinking about the consequences. Do you prefer to have chicken and spinach instead of pizza? Probably not. But if it's what you should do to reach your goal, then do it. Remember, you have the innate willpower within you just waiting for you to rouse it from its sleep. That strength will be your best ally. So stop talking about your plans and start taking action.

THE ENEMY: BOREDOM

Whenever I'm busy doing something I'm passionate about, I forget about food altogether. But if I'm bored at home, inevitably I start thinking about a glass of *atole* or an *arepa* with cheese or those "animal-style" fries from In-N-Out that I shouldn't eat. Because when I was a boy, I'd eat when I was bored. It's not that I was hungry, but I had nothing to do. If I heard the ice cream truck go by, I'd want ice cream. Or if I walked by a bakery, I'd want a treat. My life was school, homework, or sitting at my dad's job, which I found more boring than snail races. So I turned to food. And then if we went to a party, how did we celebrate? With food, of course!

Part of our Latin culture is not just eating out of boredom, but to get together and eat and drink at one another's house, laughing and dancing and singing, and, yes, even gossiping. That makes us feel like we're part of something greater than us, a community. That's just how we are raised. But my challenge to you is to change your habits. Instead of sitting on the couch watching television and surfing the web while you eat, find some outdoor activity to keep you busy. Get a group together and go for a walk or a run. Take your family to the park and play ball or some kind of board game. Not only will you replace bored eating with a family activity, but you'll also create some wonderful memories. Pick one of those activities and when you find yourself thinking about food just because you're bored, make a plan to do them. Change that habit of eating out of boredom and choose an activity that is aligned with your goal. Having that option not only keeps you from eating, but it also helps you do things that better your mind and health when you're bored.

Another way to eliminate boredom is to feed your passion, whether it's playing an instrument, writing, singing, learning a new language, acting, cooking, starting your own business, etc. And if you don't have a passion, find a fun pastime like dancing, swimming, walking, going to the museum, painting, teaching—whatever entertains you. When you're doing something that's fun or that you're passionate about, time flies. When you focus on your passion or a fun activity, you forget about everything else for a while, including that piece of leftover churro in your refrigerator, which you no doubt would have eaten if you had been bored at home.

Lastly, surround yourself with people who help you fight the boredom that leads you to eat; people who understand you, who support you, who inspire you to make choices that lead you down the right path.

YOU ARE WHO YOUR FRIENDS ARE

Often, when we want to make a major change in our lives, we don't think about how important it is to consider our social circles. We all make large and small changes in our lives, but no matter how common it is, change is hard for us. We are full of habits and rituals and routines, and if you're trying to make a change that doesn't jibe with your social group, instead of support, you might encounter resistance. It's just this simple: When we're chubby and we spend time around other chubby people, the choices we make at restaurants usually involve higher calories than what we might choose at a table full of people leading a healthy lifestyle. It happens to me. What about you?

It's very different sitting down to dinner with a group of people ordering the fattiest, greasiest, most delicious things on the menu than with people who are ordering salads. The salad eaters are going to make you think twice about ordering that hamburger. Maybe even a little guilty. And that makes us take a moment to think harder about our order. But the ones ordering burgers are going to encourage you to join them, and so you go along. It's like that with everything. If you're fighting depression and you're surrounded by people who are constantly depressed, your social circle won't be able to give you the support and inspiration you need to dig out of that sadness. They don't do it on purpose. They simply don't have it in them because they are battling those emotions, too. So you have to spread your wings and find your own way. I'm not saying you have to leave behind your old social circle. But if you find they are not helping you, you have to find at least one new friend who is willing to support and inspire you to make the changes you yearn for in your life.

Dealing with your social circle can be challenging. You might be feeling lonely and sad, you're carrying around physical and emotional weight, and the only thing you really want is to feel loved and supported. But they may offer this love through food. What to do? You're afraid to look for new people to add to your social group and be rejected, but the friends you have now aren't helping you, either. You don't know how to tell these people who care about you and want to comfort you with food that they shouldn't do that because you are afraid that they'll abandon you. Your fear of being alone makes you complacent, you say yes to everything they offer you, and slowly you start drifting further and further away from your goals. There are other alternatives. If you're willing to look for them, you can find them. Surround yourself with people who support and inspire you to create new, healthy habits that will last a lifetime.

> *Surround yourself with people who support and inspire you to create new, healthy habits that will last a lifetime.*

CREATE LASTING, HEALTHY HABITS

If you're about to take an extra bite of food and fall back into your old ways, ask yourself:

- Why do I want to eat this? Am I hungry? No.
- Am I going to eat because I feel sad or anxious? Yes.
- So why am I doing this?

That plate of food isn't going to ease your sadness. That emotion will return the second you swallow the last bite. This is one of the hardest emotional habits to break because we're too accustomed to linking food to how we feel. We learn this message as children and we're bombarded with it as we grow up. On Facebook and Instagram, our friends post all kinds of food porn photos or memes that link feelings and food. Wherever you look, that's the message you receive. We even have a term for it in English: comfort food.

> *How do we separate food from our emotions when society is teaching us the exact opposite?*

So how do we separate food from our emotions when society is teaching us the exact opposite? The idea is to attack the very moment you're about to go looking for something to eat and replace it with an activity that is good for you and doesn't involve ingesting anything. If you do it several times, you'll train your brain and you'll change your habit. You'll replace it with something healthy and manage to untether the relationship between emotion and food. Plus, you'll establish a new, healthy habit. They say that to create a new habit, you have to repeat it for at least three weeks. So stay on track for twenty-one days and you'll not only create a new habit, but you'll be making it last. And, as always, don't give up if you slip back into the old habit of eating emotionally. Don't punish yourself for it. Simply take stock of what you've done and get right back on track. We're human. It happens to all of us. What's important is not to punish yourself, but to be patient and understanding with yourself, correct the action, and keep moving forward.

DON'T BE AFRAID TO ASK FOR HELP

If you feel like all this advice isn't working and you feel stuck in a quagmire, then please, don't be afraid to ask for help. We all need assistance at some point in our lives. Helping someone and allowing yourself to be helped is one of the most beautiful things a human being can do; it's nothing to be ashamed of. Often, after we've asked for a helping hand, we realize that we just needed a little push to get us moving in the right direction. The faith and support we get from someone else us can be the first step toward making us feel better.

> *Helping someone and allowing yourself to be helped is one of the most beautiful things a human being can do.*

I know how you feel. Sometimes, you just get fed up with carrying around all this excess baggage, feeling bad all the time, and being so tired of life that you don't know what to do. That's when you need to ask for help. It's important to be able to share what you're feeling and thinking, and to let someone offer you a hand to get back on your feet and keep walking toward your goal.

That person can be a psychologist, a life coach, a mentor, a family member, a friend, a colleague, a support group, an organization, a Yes You Can! coach. Reach out to the person or organization closest to you. That support can be the key to lighting your way toward your maximum potential.

Don't let your problems sink you or make you feel cursed. There's always a way out. Hope and faith are your best allies. And if you can't see the way out clearly, ask for help. Yes You Can! has a support group, a huge family so that you never have to feel alone while you're dieting. Because I know how important it is to feel like an entire community has your back and believes in you when you feel like you can't take another step.

> *There's always a way out. Hope and faith are your best allies. And if you can't see the way out clearly, ask for help.*

Asking for help shows that you do have willpower, that you have the desire to succeed, and you want to do everything you can to achieve your goal. That call could even save your life, so don't hesitate to ask for help, please.

THE RESULT OF TAKING ACTION

While I was going through my bankruptcy in Los Angeles, working at El Pollo Loco during the week and playing a clown for kids' birthday parties on the weekends, it was actually my father who inspired me to take action. It happened one night when I had been up crying and wrestling with my life. I felt like I was beaten, like I couldn't go on. The next morning, I staggered out of bed and, with nothing to eat in the fridge, I called my father collect—because I had no money left on my cell. He picked up and I finally told him something I had been ashamed to admit before: that I'd lost my acting job and had to declare bankruptcy. That I was broke and working as a clown and at a restaurant. I told him I had $240 to my name and was carrying around a $15,000 debt.

"I don't know what to do, Dad. I don't have the strength to go on. I've kept it from you for a while now, but I can't do it anymore. What do I do? Should I write a screenplay and cast myself in it so that someone can discover my talent? But what should I even write about?"

"Why don't you tell your story?" he said.

"C'mon, Dad, who wants to read about a little fat kid from a small town in the middle of nowhere?"

"You have an incredible story that could inspire a lot of people," he insisted.

"Don't be ridiculous. You're just saying that because you're my dad."

My dad is young, so we've always been close and able to talk straight. We've gone through a lot together; he has tried to change with me over the years and I with him. We respect each other a lot, and a really nice friendship has always existed.

"I'm looking at it objectively," he told me. "Let me do this: I'm going to send you a box with a bunch of your things because I think that when you go through them, it might inspire you and give you some new ideas. This is a time for you to reflect. And you can always come home for a little while until you find your path again."

That last offer wasn't an option for me. Actually, it had made me upset to even hear him mention it, to the point that sometimes I had hung up the phone in frustration. But I was open to the other idea of him sending me a box of mementos, which, until that moment, I had blocked from my mind. When I left Maturín for Caracas, it's not just that I started a new chapter, I started an entire new *book* of my life. I closed the previous one and left everything behind. I wanted to erase it from my mind with the intent of starting a new life I could love. I'd shoved that fat little boy in that box and had forgotten about him for years. Or rather, I had *wanted* to forget about him.

That's why none of my colleagues or new friends knew about my battle with obesity, not in Caracas, not in Miami, nor in Texas or Los Angeles. If anything, I was known as the guy with the abs, the *telenovela* star; no one knew everything I'd suffered to get to that point. It never even occurred to me to mention it. Who really cared that I had lost 150 pounds? Back then, no one was posting pictures of themselves and what they were eating on Instagram . . . Instagram didn't even exist! Dieting was something you did in secret rather than sharing it with the whole world. I carried around the story of the overweight little boy from that little town, and it had formed who I was. I had buried that part of me. But one cannot completely block, forget, or deny one's past. We have to identify it, understand it, and incorporate it into our lives so we can live in peace.

When I opened the box my father sent me, I found my childhood diary, my sketch pads, my XXL graduation shirt signed by my classmates, pictures—an entire past that, until that point, I had tried to compartmentalize. But the moment I started taking out each item, the pieces of the puzzle of that scared, hurt, sad, and angry boy started to emerge. And the adult Alejandro found himself face-to-face with the boy he had tried to forget for so long. The chubby little boy inside me awoke and I thought, *Wow, this was* me. *This was my reality.* I realized at that moment that no matter how much I tried to deny it, I would never be able to silence him, because he is part of me, of my soul, of my story.

Until that moment, I hadn't realized that both could exist at the same time: the young buck who had fought for and achieved his dreams and the helpless, scared, fat little boy. I started to understand that the person I was at that point, without acknowledging who I had been, was someone I had invented. That little boy is and will always be a part of me. He's part of my DNA and partly responsible for everything I've done. I thought he was dead and buried that October 27 years ago, but the truth is he was always with me, silently. I had simply forgotten about him, dimmed him, disconnected him from my present. But he was still here.

When I started looking at the pictures my dad had sent, something unexpected happened. The anger that fat little boy had inspired in me, that he had ruined my youth—my life—was no longer there. I looked at him now with detachment and what I saw was a victim of circumstance. I scanned the pictures and thought, *That little boy was so sad.* I was smiling in every picture, but I had these sad eyes. In every picture, I was standing behind someone so you couldn't see how heavy I was. I wasn't even doing it consciously; I instinctively reacted at the sight of the camera. I had become used to avoiding them. Unconsciously, I was ashamed of my body, of who I was.

But as I looked through that box, I started to discover who I was, where I'd come from, and I finally started to understand where my fears came from. The fear of being alone. Of being abandoned. In many of the pictures, I'm eating—covering over so much of that pain I didn't even know I had, since I didn't realize my life could be any different. And then there was the school shirt. Obviously I recognized the names and that it was my shirt, but seeing it again at almost twenty-seven years old, in this new life that I'd invented, it seemed foreign to me. I was stunned to look at that XXL and realize it had been mine. How many times had I struggled to button that shirt?

While reading what my classmates had written on my shirt, I came across the names of two of my close friends who had both died in 2006 in separate car accidents, but I hadn't been able to attend their funerals because I was shooting a *telenovela*. That's when all my emotional weight clicked. I realized all I had missed out on by trying to cover up my past, to deny it: I hadn't wanted to deal with the emotions that caused everything. The new me had even forgotten about some of my best friends. A wave of sadness came over me. Seeing all these things made me understand everything I had lived through, things I had forgotten because I'd always been so focused on looking ahead and running toward the future. Yes, it's important to look forward, but we should never forget what we've learned. Our past makes up part of who we are. Instead of trying to erase or bury our past, we must accept it. We shouldn't live in the pain of past or the anxiety of the future; balance lies in living in the present. And we'll talk more about that in the next chapter.

When I looked at the pictures of me at school, I can't tell you all the emotions they stirred up in me. I saw images in the cafeteria and the hallways and I remembered all the taunts I'd suffered there. I remembered my schoolmates would stand on either side of me as I walked down the hallway and then push or taunt me as I walked by. The hallway of terror, I used to call it. Often, I just stayed in my classroom during breakfast so I wouldn't have to face that torment. How that chubby little boy suffered eating alone on the benches at school by himself. When I saw a picture of my dad's store, the first thing that came to mind was how the boy from across the street would yell out, "Hey, fatso! Better watch out, piggy! December's Christmas pig roast is right around the corner."

That box brought back so many memories and emotions that I felt I had to get them down on paper. At first, I thought about writing a screenplay, but when I sat down at my computer, I found myself writing a book. I'd never written anything professionally before, but in those pages I vented about everything that was going on inside me. All the emotions and the pain I could no longer hide from. I would stop, look at the photos again, and continue writing with tears in my eyes. I thought, *That poor, little fat boy. He had to suffer through so much at such a young age.*

I continued writing in all of my free time. At times, I had to step away because the emotions were too overwhelming. At others, I suddenly had an overwhelming urge to eat the kind of food I was having during that time, but I resisted. I'd stop, write, sleep for a few hours. And then went back to writing.

I googled how to write a book and got the idea to buy a recorder, so I could capture my thoughts before I set them down on the page. It was the perfect tool for me. I went down to the closest Radio Shack and bought the cheapest digital recorder I could afford, since I was basically broke. That way, I could record everything as it came to mind. I couldn't believe everything I had stored up in the organic hard drive of my brain. During my lunch break at El Pollo Loco, I'd get a rush of thoughts and I'd record them so I wouldn't forget them. And when I arrived at home, I would transcribe it all, and little by little, the book started coming together.

When I was far enough along with the book, I wrote to Carlos Fraga, who had published some fifteen books at that point, and asked him about an editor. He put me in touch with someone in Argentina and we got to work on it. I didn't have the money to pay him up front so we worked out a deal where I would pay him in installments.

Although I wanted to tell my entire story at first, I decided the focus should be on using the message in my story as a way of helping people live a healthier life, transform their lives, and change their bodies. When I realized how important emotional weight is and how sinisterly it can embed itself in our lives, I had to write about it. Apart from nutrition, exercise, and natural supplements, emotional health is fundamental to keeping a "happiness diet" so that you can slim your inner chubby self and transform your life forever.

In any case, I continued working as a clown and at El Pollo Loco while dedicating all my free time to the book and working with the editor. I even found a graphic designer on Craigslist who charged me just $140 to illustrate the book. (I sold my iPod to pay for it.) The entire process was a gift from God. Instead of wallowing in sadness and depression over everything that had happened to me when I went home to my lonely studio at night, I flipped on my computer and put my energy into my book. I started to transform myself from victim to victor. Once I'd expunged all the emotional weight from my soul and understood the source of my pain, I felt I had to share my story to help others going through similar circumstances. I wanted others to know that they are not alone since I knew too well what it's like to suffer that emptiness by myself.

I spent weeks and weeks dedicated to the book. By the time I moved to Miami and started doing the press rounds to promote *Eva Luna*, I realized that was the perfect time to publish my book. I printed fifteen copies through Amazon.com. I set up a Wordpress blog with a help of a friend with a link to Amazon.

Meanwhile, I was invited to be interviewed on the Spanish television show *Don Francisco Presenta* by the host of *Sábado Gigante*. I couldn't believe it. As someone who had dreamed of working in television, being asked to be on Don Francisco's show was like hitting it out of the park. It was a dream come true. Back when I used to watch that show at home in Maturín, I remember thinking that if you made it onto Don Francisco's show, it was because you were an established star. It's the show we watched together as a family every week, the one that always made that chubby little boy smile.

The day I went on the show and found myself sitting next to Don Francisco, I was super excited but also quite relaxed. I talked about the new *telenovela*, as I was expected to, but I also brought along a copy of the book. It was the first time I had publicly spoken about my past as an obese person. Wow, it was such a gratifying and important moment in my life. I watched that clip again recently and I was surprised to see how calmly I was talking about my obesity. I explained everything with such ease that it was clear I had found my calling. It was the beginning of what would become my life's purpose.

I went home that night absolutely floating on a cloud. I felt actualized, complete. I immediately called my parents to share my joy. "Did you watch me, Dad? Did you see me, Mom? Are you proud of me?" It was such a glorious moment. When I hung up, I checked my Amazon account and found that I had sold 2,700 copies of my book! The book I'd written during one of the most difficult moments in my life was actually reaching the people I'd hoped to help. It was the moment I felt I was discovering my reason for living. I was doing something no one else had done in our Latin community. It was clear my beloved Hispanic audience was starving for more of this kind of information and I was overjoyed at being able to share what I had learned. The kernel of the idea for my diet was sprouting in my heart and mind.

After that interview, I realized the power of our personal stories, of our truth, of our experiences. All I heard around town was, "Hey, Alejandro, thanks for sharing your story. I went through the same thing . . . my son is going through the same thing . . . my wife is struggling with being overweight . . ." "Chabán, you're chubby people's guardian angel." "You're the kid who used to be obese and lost all that weight, right?" Opening up my heart and telling my story to the whole world gave me the chance to connect directly with others. I was also learning how to communicate through other media. Now during interviews, instead of just asking me about the new *telenovela*, they wanted to know more about my personal story. They wanted to see photos and know all about what I had lived through. Plus it came just as *People en Español's* 50

Most Beautiful People edition hit the newsstands, and that contrast just made my story of overcoming obesity that much more impactful.

It was such a positive experience that I thought, *What can I do to continue inspiring all those people who, like me, want to change their lives but don't know how?* It became my new goal. My resolve and energy suddenly focused onto a task that brought me such satisfaction and joy. I felt like I was going from being just another actor with a book to someone with a purpose and mission that was both clear and specific. It wasn't about my ego anymore. The key question now was how could I help others. I thanked God that I could be a medium by letting my story help those around me. My life story was becoming one of hope. The book *De gordo a galán* helped open the door to my career as a motivational speaker, and with people's incredibly positive reaction to the book, I found my true calling. The chubby little boy inside me helped me find my destiny.

LIFE REWARDS ACTION

Action enables us to transform the invisible into the visible. Good things don't just fall out of the sky. Without action, there's no success. I dedicated all my Saturdays to writing this book. Often, I passed up going out with my friends on the weekends because I knew the next day I wouldn't be in any condition to exercise, write, and edit. These were all conscious decisions I made based on my desire to reach my short-term, medium-term, and long-term goals. I stayed focused and that's why I achieved what I set out to do. I often hear people finish a phrase by saying, "God willing." Now, I have a strong faith in God, and I know that at the end of the day, His will will be done because He knows what's best for us. But I also know He can't do anything for us if we aren't willing to help ourselves. Just saying "God willing" won't help us achieve what we want in life. Everything requires effort, action, desire, and perseverance. I want to emphasize "perseverance," because starting something is much harder than finishing it. Perseverance is a huge part of being successful.

> *Action enables us to transform the invisible into the visible.*

People compare themselves to me in a lot of ways and say, "Wow, you've really accomplished a lot," or "Hey, how were you able to grow your company so quickly?" "Chabán, you came to this country without knowing how to speak English and look at you now." "Chabán, you've managed to keep the weight off. Lucky you!" Friends, I promise you, magic and luck have nothing to do with what I've been able to achieve. It's all about action, effort, perseverance, and patience in my day-to-day life. God rewards hard work. It's why I wake up at 3:30 a.m. to go to work. Why, after working at *Despierta América*, I head to my Yes You Can! office and continue working. Why I work on the weekends when I run out of time during the week. Why I'm working on my other projects, like this book, my conferences, and my new Yes You Can! products instead of going out and partying. There is nothing wrong with partying, mind you. But to get ahead and reach your goals, you have to commit yourself to hard work and dedication.

If you're not willing to pay the price and sacrifice to reach your goals, then change your goals to something you can achieve. Maybe it's a less ambitious goal, maybe you won't reach what you truly want, but if you're not willing to do what it takes to reach your dream, you simply won't achieve it. Success in life isn't measure by what you achieve, but by the obstacles you overcome. Remember, success only happens when your dreams are greater than your excuses. Creating healthy and lasting habits to reach your goals isn't easy. But the benefits are worth it because these are changes that will positively change all aspects of your life.

It's normal to feel afraid. Our brain is wired to feel fear, which is what has allowed us to survive throughout the ages and protects us from pain. If fear is what's stopping you, then you have to confront that fear and give your mind, body, and spirit the green light to keep moving forward toward happiness. If anger is what's stopping you, then think before you act. Taking action requires willpower, patience, and perseverance. If you get a major craving for a Frappuccino at four in the afternoon, replace that craving with a protein shake. Also, get in touch with your inner chubby self and ask yourself if you are actually hungry or if you are turning to food for emotional reasons. If it's because you're stressed or anxious, then try to distract your mind and remind yourself of your commitment to yourself. Reread your goals, repeat your affirmation, take a look at your vision board. If you're bored, then focus on something you're passionate about. You'll soon see that if you entertain yourself doing something you love, time flies and you'll forget all about your craving.

Instead of letting the chubby voice inside you talk about the things you want to eat—cake or pie or nachos covered in cheese—try to change that internal dialogue into something more positive. Think of something you love to do, something to take your mind off the craving. Visualize how you want to look when you overcome that craving and lose the weight that's keeping your from reaching your goal. I'll bet that after a couple of minutes, you'll have forgotten about your craving. Remember, the goal is to replace your negative habits with positive ones until they become a healthy way of life. Keep practicing until it becomes the new norm in your life.

I find that these days when I'm under stress or feeling anxious or am in pain, that's when I eat the best. It's a challenge; I want to look better. If I suffer a breakup, instead of running and eating everything in the fridge, I run to my bike and get the stress out in a way that's working toward my goal. However, getting to the point where I don't just fall into bed and cry and eat out of control took years. It was a conscious decision I made a long time ago. I also learned that instead of playing the part of the victim, I should follow the path of the victor. But you have to put that into practice and keep working without giving up. These 7 steps have been a sort of happiness diet. When my life feels out of balance, knowing that I at least can control what I eat and how I take care of my body helps me reestablish that balance.

> *Don't make your decisions lightly.*
> *Analyze them carefully. Map out your strategy.*
> *And then take action.*

Don't make your decisions lightly. Analyze them carefully. Map out your strategy. And then take action. If you want to get from the couch to the door, you have to get up and walk there. You're not going to float there by magic. Similarly, don't wait for success to fall out of the sky without putting forth any effort. Get up and start working toward the changes you want to see in your life. Don't limit yourself and don't let yourself get stuck. I know you can accomplish so much more than you think. As I always say, intention plus action leads to results. You have greatness within you and I know you can reach a higher level and overcome any challenge before you—even those that seem insurmountable. You are a gladiator. You are made in the image of God, designed to succeed. That magnificent strength is within you. Remember, if you've made it this far, you can go even further. Yes You Can!

Essential tips to transform your life

- Don't take your decisions lightly. Analyze them with your goals in mind, since each decision affects the next.

- Disarm that enemy called boredom by empowering your passions and interests instead of your stomach.
- Distance yourself from negative people and surround yourself with people who support and inspire you to make new and lasting habits.
- Take action to achieve your goals. Without action, there is no movement.

Put It into Practice!

TAKE ACTION

One action leads to another. Having the willpower to put your plan into motion, to take that first step, even to ask for help, is so much more important than you can imagine. So today, right now, I want you to do something that will help get you closer to your goal.

- If your goal is to buy a house, today, instead of buying your usual Starbucks coffee, take that money and put it into an envelope labeled "Savings for My New Home."
- If your goal is to get angry less often, today I want you to go out of your way to say something nice to someone.
- If your goal is to get a new job, I want you to go on the Internet right now and do a search, or work on your résumé, or make a call to one person who can give you solid advice about what you need to do next.
- If your goal is to lose weight, right now, go throw out every bit of junk food in your house and go to the supermarket and buy something healthy instead, like leafy greens, proteins, or fresh fruit.

Although your goal may seem far away, each step you take toward it gets you that much closer. And the more steps you take in that direction, the faster you'll reach your goal. So congratulate yourself right now for the *action* you have taken today to get you closer to your goal. Tomorrow, do it again. If you've made it this far, you can go even further. I believe in you!

María José Escalante

My name is María José Escalante. I was born in El Salvador, and by age seven, I was already obese and suffered from high cholesterol. When I moved to the United States, I gained even more weight. My whole young life, I'd look in the mirror and hate who I saw staring back at me. I'd grab my stomach and say to myself, "You make me so unhappy. I hate you!" My mother would see how sad I was and would take me for ice cream to help me feel better. Everyone around me said, "You're never going to lose weight because you're just big boned and this is your natural constitution."

I tried to kill myself with sleeping pills twice because I didn't want to live this nightmare of weighing 221 pounds. Depression and isolation made me want to eat more and more. I kept trying to calm my emotions with food.

One day my mother told me about Alejandro Chabán's program, and I informed her, "That can't be true. Those people haven't been fat their whole lives like me." After some convincing, I decided to give Yes You Can! a try.

I started to love the vegetables in the diet manual and I began choosing better carbohydrates. In eight months, I dropped sixty pounds. I went from a size XXL to a medium. My whole life changed. Now at twenty-three years old, I feel like God has a plan for me and that it's my calling to inspire others with optimism and my story! I'm finally happy. Yes You Can!

SUCCESS STORY

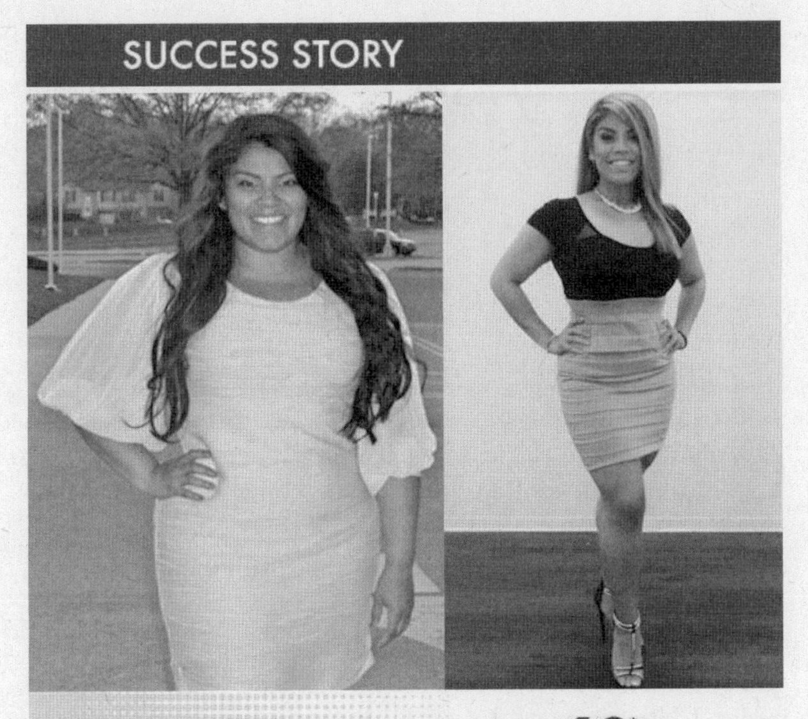

MARÍA JOSÉ ESCALANTE lost 60* lbs

MARÍA JOSÉ'S ADVICE: *What helped me was keeping my fat clothes as a reminder of where I'd been, what I'd overcome, and how much I'd fought to reach this weight—and how badly I never want to slip back there again.*

**Results not typical and will vary according to diet, exercise, metabolism, and genetic makeup.*

⟨ TEN ⟩

Step 7: Focus on the Present

CONGRATULATIONS! YOU'VE ARRIVED at the seventh and final step to healing your soul! I'm so happy to know you're here, reading this final chapter and soaking in all this advice. I hope this experience will help heal you from the inside out, just as you deserve. Now, let's get to work!

First a confession: This final step is one I still work on every day, the one that is the hardest for me, the one I sometimes forget. It's not because I don't understand how important it is. Rather my desire to reach my goal sometimes overwhelms the need to enjoy, give thanks, and live in the present. So often we focus so much on our goals and achieving them that we forget to enjoy the journey.

> *Depression is an excess of the past.*
> *Anxiety is an excess of the future.*
> *Peace is living in the moment.*

Today is a gift from God—that's why we call it the present. It's the place where we can both dream and take action. It's the moment when we can give thanks for everything that has happened and all that will come. The key is finding the right balance to not lose ourselves in the past or the future. Not too long ago, I came across a meme on social media that perfectly captured this final step we're about to explore: *Depression is an excess of the past. Anxiety is an excess of the future. Peace is living in the moment.* I couldn't have said it better myself. That's what I want for you, for myself, for everyone: for us to live in peace and harmony, fighting for our dreams but enjoying the journey.

DON'T LET THE PAST OR FUTURE RUN YOUR LIFE

Why do people say that good things happen when you least expect them? Because when you wait for them, you're living in the future. You create expectations and that disconnects you from the reality of the present. That doesn't mean you shouldn't be proactive and work toward your goals. Do your work, value today, and leave the rest to God. Be thankful for TODAY. Don't hold on to the past. Appreciate the NOW.

Focusing on the past or the future allows those to take total control over your life and it alienates you from the present. The past pulls you back, turns you into a victim of circumstances, and makes you remember what was. And it makes you think, "Oh, poor me," or "If only I had . . ." You have to learn to let go of that weight and keep one fundamental truth clear in your mind: The past only served to turn you into who you are today. The past was and always will be part of your life, part of your lessons. Remember, you may not be able to change the past, but you can do something in the present to change the future. It's an important part of who you are today. You shouldn't try to erase your past because there is no way to escape it.

> *Remember, you may not be able to change the past, but you can do something in the present to change the future.*

If you erased the errors in your past, you'd end up erasing all the wisdom in your present. What you need to do is study your past, accept it, and forgive it. In the words of the great Paulo Coelho: "Forgiving your past is giving your future a chance." You are creating your future in the present. It's all about balance and how you decided to tell your story today. If you're constantly referring to the past and tying it to the present, you'll never be able to move on. You'll remain anchored to yesterday without being able to enjoy what is happening right now. The key to managing your past is to realize that what happened was not necessarily your fault and that the circumstances in your life also played a role in what happened. You have to understand there were things you couldn't control, things that were out of your hands. But if you can take responsibility for how you feel today, then you can change what your past means to you.

Recently, I had a moment when I was taken back to the past and I relived some of those same emotions. It made me realize what a waste of time it is to cling to the events of yesterday. It's all about perspective. I had traveled to Puerto Rico to launch some new Yes You Can! products. Afterward, a young man from the audience came up to me and said, "Chabán, hey, it's me!" He was a bald, overweight man about my age. At first, I honestly didn't recognize him, until he was right in front of me and said his name. My heart stopped. It turned out to be one of my Maturín classmates—one of the cruelest kids in the class. One of the ones who made me suffer the most. The tall, skinny kid from my memory was now standing in front of me, saying hello as if nothing had happened. I couldn't believe it.

I shook his hand, feeling a tsunami of emotions, thinking, *Should I spit in his face? Punch his lights out?* I didn't, but I had the urge. We talked a bit and he told me he had come to the event to personally ask me for advice on losing weight. *This bastard who had made my life hell when I was fat was now asking me for help?* I was stunned, but I took the opportunity to say to him:

"Sure, I'd love to go to lunch because we have a lot to talk about. You hurt me so much that I'd like the chance to sit down with you and heal those old wounds."

"I hurt you?" he asked.

I couldn't understand his reaction, yet he was so genuinely surprised. I said goodbye to my team and went off to have lunch with him. When we finally sat down, I told him the truth.

"I'm glad we're sitting down to lunch because it's important for me to close this chapter of my life," I said, and told him about my experience in high school. "Most of the times when I was hurting and crying the most, it was because of something you had done. You called me names. You called me a fat, greasy *arepa*. You have no idea how much damage that caused me."

I had no idea what he was going to say. I had no idea what to expect from this encounter, but I knew I had to express myself fully and get this pain and anguish out once and for all. I never would have expected his response.

"Alejandro, bud, I'm sorry, but I don't remember any of that," he said, looking stunned, tears in his eyes.

I had carried around all this pain, this hate, for all these years and he didn't even remember. That's perspective for you. To him, it was a joke he'd made in the moment and almost immediately forgot about it. Meanwhile, to me, his words were a daily torture I took home that caused me to break down in the silence and solitude of my room. I thought he hated me and I didn't know why. If he was in the cafeteria, I wouldn't even go in because I knew he would make fun of me. If he was in one of my classes, I'd make sure to come in late. This person had played such a pivotal role in my life and my daily decisions back then, and now I came to find out that he didn't even remember any of it. It was a huge lesson.

That conversation and realization made me feel both relieved and furious at myself at the same time. I couldn't believe I had let myself carry around so much pain and anger for so many years and that it had kept me from fully enjoying my adolescence. I felt so helpless at learning he didn't even remember that entire episode in my life. I asked myself, "Why did I give that so much importance?" I felt so stupid. At the same time, it helped me understand his side of the story. During our conversation, he told me that during that time his parents were going through a divorce and things were tough at home. He learned that the more trouble he got into at school, the more attention he would get, because his mother would come to school to get him. It was how he maintained a connection with her, however brief. So he kept doing it over and over because as children, that's the only way we know to get attention.

Hearing his words, his perspective, opened my eyes. It served as a reminder of how many things someone else might be going through behind the scenes. Sometimes those who hurt us aren't necessarily trying to do us damage but rather they are going through some kind of suffering themselves. Everyone has his or her own story. That's why there are so many cases of children who beat up or abuse other children and we later come to find out that's the way they are being treated at home. They've learned to use their fists and harsh words as communication tools because no one in their lives has shown them otherwise. I learned so much that day. It turned out to be a wonderful encounter. What started out as a conversation to make peace ended up becoming so much more.

Now it's your turn. Now you have to decide whether you want to continue being a victim of your past or overcome it in the present. It's in your hands whether you want to take the time to look at the pain of your earlier years and examine what is causing your emotional weight. I want you to understand it's not something you chose, but it happened to you anyway. Now it's up to you to decide how you'll feel about that situation: You can stay stuck in a moment forever, like some kind of martyr, saying poor me, or you can transform that pain into something that prompts you to learn from the situation and grow from it. Turn it in your favor. Ask yourself the following:

- What positive came from that situation?
- What can I learn or extract from those painful experiences so I can evolve today?
- How can this help me?

Now do the following exercise to begin freeing yourself from your past and focusing on the present.

Put It into Practice!

LEARN TO FORGIVE

Is there someone from your past who still haunts your memories? Someone who affects your present, who makes you feel rage or sadness or frustration at the memory? Someone you feel responsible for the state of your life right now? Well, today, I want you to learn to forgive that person. How?

- *Write to him or her.* Take pen and paper or open a computer document and begin with "Dear" whoever. Write them a personal letter.
- *Express yourself.* Describe what you feel and what they made you feel. Explain how those experiences affect you to this day. Say everything you've always wanted to say, everything you rehearsed in your mind but never said out loud.
- *Forgive him or her.* Once you've expressed yourself honestly and written everything you've been holding in all this time, forgive this person. If you want to spell out everything you forgive him or her for, that's good. If you simply want to say, "I forgive you," that's more than enough.

The purpose of this letter is to free yourself from this baggage, this pain caused by a person who is no longer in your present. If it's someone you are still in contact with, you can send the letter or maybe you can get coffee with him or her and speak openly and honestly, but this isn't necessary. With the simple act of putting all this pain down on the page, you'll feel a huge relief. Repeat the words "I forgive you," once, twice, three times—as many times as necessary until you truly feel these words in your soul and you finally feel lighter and free. Congratulations! This isn't an easy exercise, but it is incredibly healing.

Living in the past, lamenting everything that was and no longer is, can only cause you sadness. And that sadness can become depression over time. Meanwhile, living in the future can cause anxiety, stress, and fear. Fear of what's to come. Fear of the unknown. Fear of success. If we free ourselves from the past but go to the other extreme and only focus on the future, that can also become toxic. Focusing on something we do not have power over, something we can't say for sure will ever come to pass, also isn't healthy because there's nothing we can do to control it. That's why the key to balance is in the present.

Don't let the ghosts of your past and the fears of the future control your life.

Don't let the ghosts of your past and the fears of the future control your life. Live in the here and now. Focus on the present. That's where you should put all your energy. Life is about living in the moment with passion and enthusiasm. Appreciate and enjoy it. Leave the past in the past, the future in the future, and live in the moment.

THE THREE PS: LIVE IN THE *PRESENT* WITH *PATIENCE* AND *PERSEVERANCE*

Whatever doesn't kill you makes you stronger. Don't let your past fears and your anxiety over the future ruin your present because the only thing that's sure in this life is birth, death, and this very moment.

As I mentioned at the beginning of this chapter, I'm still working on this step. I try to disconnect from what has happened and what will happen and instead focus on what's happening now. In this time of Instagram, Snapchat, Facebook, and Twitter, we spend our days thinking about who is happier than us, how we can impress our friends, or show our exes how much happier we are without them. You mean to tell me you've never been lying in bed on a Friday night without plans and said to yourself, "I'm going to post this picture from a few days ago so my ex or my friends see how happy I am"? Well, *I* have! Haha! On the other hand, sometimes I'm at a get-together and already thinking about the next party or project. Or I reach my goal and instead of celebrating it, I'm already thinking about the next goal. I have to make a conscious effort to stop and realize when I'm doing this. I tell myself, "Hold on, Alejandro. Enjoy the moment because this moment won't come again." For many of us who are immigrants, it's tough to focus on the present, because part of us is always thinking about our country of origin: our family who are still there, when they might come, when our immigration papers will come through, when we'll have a good enough job so we can send money back home. Our minds are filled with these thoughts, and before we know it, *poof*, we forget about the present. About the here and now.

It's fine to want to get ahead, to want to help, but to do both, first you have to focus on the present. This moment is not just for working and toiling. We have to enjoy it! We have to thank God for another day and we should take advantage of it, not just by laboring but also by enjoying the journey.

Yes, it's important to take action today so that tomorrow we can get our papers in order or so we can land that job. But let us not forget to celebrate being alive and valuing our time with our families and friends. Let us not forget to pay attention to the signals the Universe is sending us. Everything goes hand in hand.

You have to show a lot of willpower and commitment to work today toward what you hope will happen five or ten years from now. We all lose patience at one point or another. We want results *now*. We want to work hard today and immediately see the fruits of our labor. At some point, we've all wanted to lose these extra pounds immediately and we've stood on the bathroom scale, hoping it will show that we've lost the weight. But when you see your weight unchanged, you get upset and you run out to buy that girdle your friend told you about. You wear it all week and when you step on the scale you realize it didn't help at all, and you actually gained four pounds. You're frustrated and lose sleep. So you're up at night when a commercial comes on for a piece of exercise equipment that's supposed to give you buns of steel in just a few days, and you buy it without your husband knowing. You use it before anyone comes home from work so they won't laugh at you. You sweat through it for two weeks, and when you weigh yourself with great expectations, you become furious to realize you haven't lost a pound. So you go on your Facebook page and see there's a diet plan that millions of people are using and you decide to call. You speak to a Yes You Can! coach, order the packet; it arrives, but you decided to do it your way instead of the planned method. You don't read the nutritional guide because it's too long and, besides, you tell yourself you know how to diet. You begin following the plan according to your own theory. You go to your nephew's baptism and eat and drink like everyone else, and the next week, when you step on the scale, you realize you are exactly the same weight. What's going on? You say that the Yes You Can! diet didn't work for you. Have you noticed the common denominator in all this? It's not the girdle, the exercise equipment, or the plan. It's you!

You are the one who isn't assuming the responsibility of your commitment and following the steps. It all depends on you. That's why it's so important to stay focused, patient, and persistent. Every fruit needs a chance to grow and mature. The sapling you plant today must be watered regularly, and you have to have patience for it to bloom in its own time. You will have to wait all four seasons for this flower to bloom and bear fruit. And at some point, that flower also will die and give room for other buds to bloom. In the same way, your goals, once achieved, will make room for other goals and dreams. It's a circle that we must all understand, respect, and accept.

We have to keep working on ourselves, taking stock of the things that help and heal us, finding our balance, and remaining aware of this when life puts obstacles in our way. It's not about the circumstances. It's about *you*. There will always be moments in life that knock us off balance. Moments of pain and sadness, moments of frustration and rage when everything feels out of control. The key is learning to be conscious of those moments, analyze the situation, and realize how these experiences help us focus on the present. The road may be long, so enjoy the ride. Appreciate what is around you. The past is useful only when it reveals something to us about the present. The present is what matters.

MAKE PEACE WITH THE CHUBBY PERSON INSIDE YOU

I used to always compare myself to my friends and colleagues, asking them how they managed to eat everything they wanted and keep those rock-hard abs. I wanted to be like them. I was living in the future. I couldn't understand why I had been destined to be chubby and carry around all this baggage. I was living in the past. That restlessness came from by emotional weight. I hadn't yet learned to accept my inner chubby self, to forgive him, to love him, and to make peace with him so I could live in the present. I was still blaming him for all he'd made me suffer. I was still positioning myself as a victim of circumstance and everything that had happened to me. I hadn't taken responsibility. In time I realized we all have fears to confront and pain to heal.

The chubby person inside me sometimes blows up in anger if he thinks someone is trying to hurt him. It has everything to do with my past and not knowing how to deal with it because that situation takes me to my childhood pain, to that resentment, to the constant mocking. I feel like I have to be perfect to be loved, and if something doesn't go according to plan, I don't react positively.

But these days, when this happens, instead of getting angry at that part of myself, I try to talk to that part of my being and make peace with him. I've learned it doesn't help to get upset or punish myself. It only brings me bigger problems. The key is to forgive, accept, love, and make peace TODAY with that chubby person inside. We have to accept that this was the lesson we were meant to learn in life.

> *The key is to forgive, accept, love, and make peace TODAY with that chubby person inside us.*

The next time something "bad" happens to you—when you feel you've been personally attacked or unjustly treated—instead of thinking, *Why do these horrible things happen to me?*, I want you to replace it with this thought: *I'm glad this happened because I can grow and learn from life's tough experiences.* In the face of every situation you don't like, instead of asking yourself, "What's wrong?" ask yourself, "What's great?"

HOW I BECAME WHO I AM TODAY

The fact that all of you responded to my story changed my life. I felt it was like a rebirth because I suddenly saw everything with fresh eyes, from a different perspective. A whole new world I'd never imagined opened up to me. Revealing and accepting my past helped me find my new purpose in life: being a light to those around me.

As this door opened to me, I delved further into this theme. I wanted to come up with a solution for Latinos created by a Latino, a healthy option that would help our generation and the next. That's how I came to found my company, to help others not just lose weight but to establish a healthy lifestyle without abandoning their Latin roots. Over the years, I'd tried all the fad diets. I know how bad they are. I was never able to connect with their message. And I knew the reason was it felt it didn't understand me or my Latino culture.

I studied day and night. I read books, encyclopedias, websites, blogs. I interviewed doctors, nutritionists, trainers, and gastroenterologists. I was on a mission to find the best way to help people struggling with their weight. Later, I took a poster board and wrote down and pasted pictures of all the ways I wanted my story to help others. I wrote down everything about all these diets that, being from another country, had never made sense to me. I wanted to help people of all ages, backgrounds, creeds, and accents because all of us who are overweight feel the same, regardless of our stories. We all have the same heart.

While I was thinking about all this, I got the call to compete on *Mira Quién Baila (Look Who's Dancing),* but I didn't want to do it at first. I tried to explain to them that I wasn't a dancer. Between you and me, the truth is I didn't know how to dance! I didn't tell them how scared I was to be on the show. I didn't think I could measure up and I was terrified of exposing myself in that way. I didn't want to be in a situation where

I was insecure about something I didn't know how to do. My inner chubby kid rose to the surface.

When I should have learned to dance as a boy, I was too overweight and never did it. Whenever I went to family functions, I stayed seated because I was embarrassed to try to dance. Or when I went to parties with friends as an adult, I'd stay at the table or would stand idly by watching others dance. I was ashamed to try to dance and be terrible at it. After a lot of back and forth, I finally told myself, "C'mon, just do it!" And I did. I said yes and joined the *Mira Quién Baila* cast, where I was proud to represent First Lady Michelle Obama's Let's Move Foundation. I chose it because it helps young people make conscious decisions about their health. It was a great opportunity not only to overcome my fears but also to continue sharing my story with more people. I even told the story of not learning to dance because of my obesity.

I was super nervous during those first few rehearsals, dancing in front of a camera, not because I was doing good or bad, but because I was worried about what others might think. My insecurities came to the surface, those fears borne out of my emotional weight. I was scared people would make fun of me, that they would realize I didn't know how to dance, that I would fall down in the middle of the routine, that I would be the first one cut. In short, I was afraid to fail. I was exposing myself by doing something I didn't know how to do and that stirred up some old demons, which I had thought I had under control.

Moreover, I'm an uber perfectionist. So when practice would end at 5:00 p.m., I would want to stay longer, sometimes until 9:00 p.m. My whole life started revolving around the show, around my goal of not messing up. I was so concentrated on the result that I forgot to enjoy the moment. A couple years later, when I watched other episodes of the show, I thought, *I was so dumb to be so worried instead of just enjoying myself and laughing and falling without worrying so much.*

It's just that when I was overweight, my intellect was the

only thing I had going for me. People would always say, "Whoa, Chabán, you're so smart," while the titles of cool and handsome went to someone else. So during the show, I turned the reins over to my intellect when I should have just had fun. Recently, Alicia Miracles, my neurolinguistic programming therapist, pointed out something to me that really caught me off guard. She noticed that I often said I "wasn't capable" but never used the phrase "I deserve." She told me capability was linked to reason, to the intellect, but being deserving was something else entirely. To be deserving means to feel that we have value so that the things we desire have a place in our lives. She was so right. I never felt like I deserved things. But I always felt I had the capacity to achieve them. There was a disconnect between my mind and soul.

That experience underscored how important it is to enjoy the journey and to feel like we deserve good things in our lives. Sure, we have to stay focused on our goal, but we should not let that override the joy in the moment. Because if we don't allow ourselves to feel joy during the process, it becomes a painful, arduous journey where instead of ridding ourselves of excess baggage, we actually take on more.

We have to learn to take the things that happen to us in stride.

We have to learn to take the things that happen to us in stride. Sometimes we'll fall. Sometimes things won't go the way we hope. But when this happens, we simply need to get up, learn from the experience, and keep moving forward. We have to learn to forgive ourselves. We all make mistakes. But we shouldn't keep punishing ourselves for that for the rest of our lives. We have to learn to forgive the mistakes we've made, learn from our past, and keep moving ahead with a smile.

In the end, I finished fourth on *Mira Quién Baila*. I injured myself and was eliminated. The challenge taught me a very valuable lesson: We have to enjoy every moment, living in the present, because once it's over, there's no going back.

Meanwhile, every day I was getting closer to bringing forth a plan that would help provide others with a healthy lifestyle. That's how we came to create Yes You Can! I spent my days answering key questions: "What do I want to do? If I were overweight again, what would I wish I had that I didn't have back then?" That's how I began to define the plan, based on my own experiences.

A lot of people supported me and believed in me along the way. Having people who support you on your path toward happiness gives you strength just when you think you can't go any further. That push is essential, that feeling that you have a community's support cheering you on. That's why I included coaches as part of Yes You Can!, because I know how difficult it is when we don't have support at home or among our friends. And I know how important it is to have someone support you.

Having people who support you on your path toward happiness gives you strength just when you think you can't go any further.

Throughout this whole process of creating this company, sometimes I'd get frustrated at all the obstacles in my way, and I'd want to throw in the towel. With each step back—when the logo was wrong or the website name wasn't available or the supplies didn't arrive on time—I felt defeated. But these are just little tests God puts in our path and that we need to overcome. That's when we have to fight the hardest to come out ahead. That's what will make success taste that much sweeter when you reach your goal.

All of these experiences taught me over and over that things don't always turn out the way we want. We must overcome a thousand pebbles and boulders in our path, but it's always worth the effort, perseverance, and patience because it helps us understand and grow as human beings. We learn that when we love and have a passion for a dream, every sacrifice is worth it.

Today, when I walk into the huge building where Yes You Can! has its offices, my heart skips a beat, my body vibrates, and I feel like I'm standing in our temple, the place where we change lives. I give God thanks for granting me the opportunity to transform millions of lives through my experiences and mission.

IT ALL DEPENDS ON YOU

I'm convinced that you can achieve the changes you want, inside and out. You have the 7 steps in your hands. You know my story. You have other people's success stories and other anecdotes as inspirational examples for what to do and what not to do. And you have my complete faith in you. Now all that's missing is for you to have faith in yourself. Now you have to be inspired to face your own fears once and for all, heal your soul, and lose your emotional weight.

I know that by following these steps you're going to open up and heal your emotional weight, which you've been carrying around for so long. I know this will all guide you to an unlimited universe where you can achieve the physical, mental, and emotional changes that will lead you toward your biggest dreams.

Now, we have to be clear that living in the moment doesn't mean living as if there is no tomorrow. This does not mean you have every excuse to lavish every desire upon yourself today without caring about the future. This isn't the point. The present, as with your actions, affirmations, and visualizations, should also be aligned with your goals. Remember that the decisions you make today will affect your tomorrow. Focus on the present and keep an eye on the future.

The decisions you make today
will affect your tomorrow.

The most important part of this and what you should never lose sight of is GRATITUDE! Every night before I go to bed, I think about the ten things I'm grateful for. Give thanks for everything you have, everything you've experienced, everything around you. Give thanks for being alive. Without gratitude, there are no goals, no affirmations, no visualizations, or actions that are worth a damn.

The biggest gift I want you to discover in this process is that the tools to achieve the life of your dreams are within you. The history that has made you suffer is your greatest gift. I know you can achieve it. I know you'll reach whatever goal you set for yourself. Focus and go forward. You deserve it!

Essential advice to transform your life

- Don't let the past or the future run your life.
- Live in the present, acting with patience and perseverance to reach your dreams.
- Make peace with the chubby voice inside you. Forgive him. Accept him. Love him.
- Give thanks for everything in your life.
- Focus on the miracle of the present. Have faith. Have the boldness to face your fears so you can finally achieve the change, inside and outside, that you desperately desire.

Put It into Practice!

TRANSFORM THE "WHY?" INTO "FOR WHAT PURPOSE?"

To free yourself from the guilt and pain of your past so that you can take responsibility for your future and enjoy your present, you need to take action. If you're still asking "why" everything had to happen to you, I have some bad news for you: You're still living in the past. What you need to do, as we saw in Chapter 2, is replace the "why" with "for what purpose." "For what purpose did this happen to me?" Remember: Your thoughts affect your feelings and your actions.

If you ask yourself, "Why am I so poor?" your mind is automatically going to respond, "Because my parents were poor. Because I'm irresponsible. Because my husband left me. Because me ex-wife took everything." The only thing this question does is fill you with negative thoughts that only pull you back and turn you into a victim again—they take you to a place where there is no *action*.

Now, if you change the question to ask "What is the purpose of my being poor?" this leads you to ask how you can learn from the situation or circumstance. The answers you'll find will be, "So that I can understand what it means to be poor. So that I can value when I do have some money and not take it for granted. So that I can understand that material things do not validate me." When we ask "for what purpose?" we find other answers. "For what purpose did God make me fat?" For the purpose of teaching you a lesson, so that you can help others overcome this obstacle. Purge "why" from your vocabulary and replace it with "for what purpose," and stop living in the past. It's time to use yesterday's lessons to understand today. If you ask better questions, you'll arrive at better answers.

Ludi Ordoñez

My name is Ludi Ordoñez and I'm twenty-eight years old. I live in my beautiful Guatemala. My childhood was very traumatic because of my alcoholic father, who made my home life chaos. My only refuge from the violence and yelling was food, candy, and chocolate. I protected myself with a layer of fat.

I was surrounded by taunts and humiliation at school. To my classmates, I didn't have a name. I was just "Fat Girl." They'd pretend like they were going to hug me and then laugh in my face, saying no one's arms were long enough to wrap all the way around my 260 pounds.

I always felt isolated. I never had a boyfriend as a teen. And if my obesity wasn't bad enough, weight gain actually cost me one of the most important people in my life: my sister. She died suddenly from not being able to breathe because of her obesity. This loss made me eat even more. I hated myself and kept eating until I was a size 3XL.

But soon after her death, I decided I needed to lose weight. When I heard Alejandro Chabán's story, I felt like I wasn't alone, that there was someone who understood my suffering. With Yes You Can!, I felt like someone was with me every day, my new family. I realized there was a light at the end of the tunnel.

Today, after ten months, I have lost 120 pounds and I've managed to keep it off for six months and counting. I regained the will to live. I found love and I am the woman of my dreams. I can. You can. Yes You Can!

SUCCESS STORY

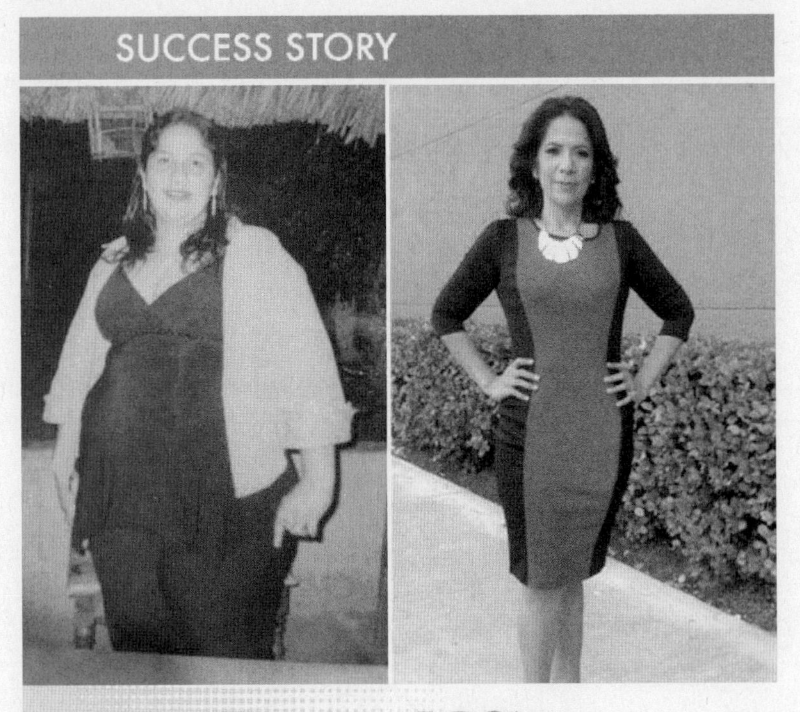

LUDI ORDOÑEZ **lost 120* lbs**

LUDI'S ADVICE: *What helped me the most was changing my attitude, thinking that this* was *going to work. And I wouldn't let anyone tell me otherwise. If my family told me it wasn't going to work, that I was going to get sick, I showed them otherwise. Another thing that helped was planning out my meals. That way, I had no excuses.*

**Results not typical and will vary according to diet, exercise, metabolism, and genetic makeup.*

❬ PART THREE ❭

This Is Just the Beginning!

⟨ ELEVEN ⟩

From Darkness to Light

IN THIS BOOK we have focused on how emotions relate to weight, but remember that a thin person can have emotional weight as well. The emotions that weigh on us are a reflection of the pain, loss, and sadness we have carried around since we were children. Poverty, loss, abandonment, deaths, divorces, childhood traumas—are all reflected in the decisions we make throughout our lives.

Scenarios change as we age. We move, get married, have families, migrate to other countries, change jobs, but if we don't pay attention to our emotional weight over the years, our emotional weight continues to grow—and it will follow us wherever we go. If we continue to ignore this weight on our souls, we might be able to function, but we will continue to feel as if our path is littered with boulders and challenges. And the irony is that we are the ones putting the boulders in our path. When you finally realize this, you'll feel a relief like you can't believe. All of a sudden, you'll feel so light that you will realize you can achieve any goal you set your mind to.

It's not an easy road. It takes time, patience, perseverance, and faith. But it is possible and it's wonderful. When you achieve this, celebrate it and enjoy the moment, in the present. Stop living in the past, but don't try to forget it. Now that you've become aware of your emotional weight and managed to apply the 7 steps to heal your soul, don't let any excuse lead you back to eating as an escape again. Don't drown your sorrows in food anymore. Look for alternatives. I know exactly how you feel because I've lived it. I know what it's like to take refuge in food and how dangerous it can be. And I also know what it's like to make the right choices that take us down a better path. It took me years to understand my emotional weight, where it came from and how to cure it. That's why I wrote this book, to share with you in these few pages what it took me a lifetime to understand.

Only now, looking back, can I identify the key moments when things clicked for me. The first was in Caracas. Those two and a half years I lived in the capital were essential for me because it was when I was able to finally commit to myself, focus on myself and on my career. It was the place where I began to discover the emotional weight I carried inside.

Then, a few years later in Dallas, when I started learning about body building, musculature, and anatomy, something clicked again. I started to understand the relationship between the physical and the emotional.

Then I experienced a personal trial in Los Angeles, when a devastating bankruptcy became a moment of personal growth. During this time I was inspired to write my first book, *De gordo a galán*. It was the first time I brought everything I was feeling out into the light. Only then did I finally understand what was happening to me. It was the missing piece of the puzzle. That was the moment when I truly started healing my emotional weight.

One of the last revelations came with the creation of Yes You Can! That's when I truly understood my mission in life, my reason for being. I understood why and for what purpose I was placed on earth, my commitment to God, and to all of you.

As you'll see, it's a lifelong process that starts with baby steps that evolve into much bigger ones, with short-, medium- and long-term goals. You never know when you're going to learn a new lesson and how it can become a gift to help you further understand your emotional weight. That's why I ask you to stay present, connected, and attentive to what's happening around you. Don't be afraid of your emotions. They're there to help you. They're trying to communicate something bigger to you. Pay attention to them so you can balance them before they become toxic.

> *Don't be afraid of your emotions. They're there to help you. They're trying to communicate something bigger to you.*

I continue to work on myself and will keep at it for the rest of my life, because there's always something new to learn. As a matter of fact, I recently learned a new lesson that I want to share with you. It was a realization that lightened my soul and brought me such a wonderful sensation of peace that I haven't felt in a long time. It was a moment of complete acceptance and forgiveness. It's when I finally became best friends with the overweight little boy inside me.

• • •

My relationship with the chubby little boy inside me has been evolving over the years. The road has been more like a roller coaster of emotions and feelings that I am only now beginning to understand. It all began to reveal itself on October 27, 1997, when I declared that the chubby little boy was dead. Back then, I thought I could kill him and forget about him. But later, I realized he was still inside me. So at the end of my first book, I decided to give the little boy wings and let him fly. However, after sharing my story publicly and founding Yes You Can!, I realized that the little boy would always be an essential part of my story. I didn't have to kill him or liberate him or alienate him. Rather, I had to accept him and love him. It took me eighteen years of struggle to arrive at this realization. It was only recently, in October 2015, that I learned this most valuable lesson.

I started to realize that he was dormant for many years, waking up every now and then to make me feel certain fears, insecurities, and rage, which made me understand that he lived inside my soul and could sabotage my dreams whenever he wanted to. So with the knowledge that I couldn't get rid of him, I learned to channel that rage whenever he reared his head. Every time I felt like he was going to disrupt something, I grabbed him by the ear and shook him, locked him in a dark room in my soul so he couldn't interfere with my thoughts and emotions. I wanted to show him I was boss, and he needed to stop bothering me or suffer the consequences.

One day, while I was talking to my therapist, I told her about all this and she responded with a simple but insightful question: "Does that work for you?" I told her it had worked when it came to my personal relationships but that it hadn't worked as I'd hoped in other parts of my life. "So what do you think you should do about that?" she asked. I didn't know what to answer. I'd gotten used to dealing with my inner chubby kid this way and didn't know how else to treat him.

Noticing my silence, she changed strategies and asked me this way: "In which hand would you say is the mature, successful person who has clear goals?" I waved my right hand. "And where is the chubby little boy inside you, the one who is defensive and you have to beat back into submission?" I raised my left hand. My right hand was open, relaxed, in control. My left hand, I realized, was balled up into a fist—tense, ready to defend myself. I looked down at my hands and was stunned. I couldn't believe it. Unknowingly, my emotions were reflected in my physical gesture.

I was only beginning to discover that I continued to fight with the chubby boy inside me because I felt he always interfered with the good things in my life. He made me blow up at my loved ones and even insult people I truly cared about. I only had to care about someone for my inner troubled child to come out and sabotage the relationship with the words I'd hidden behind for safety as a boy.

My therapist explained to me that the problem with my coping strategy—locking up the inner boy in the cellar and tying him to a chair to keep him from interfering—was that I was in fact abusing him. *I was abusing myself.* I was still punishing that side of myself for everything "he" had done to me. I stuffed him in a dark place and beat him up so that he would obey me and understand the man that I had become. Sure, if you intimidate someone and lock them in a room with their arms and legs tied and their mouth gagged, it works for a while. It had worked for me until then. I'd managed to control him, but it was only a temporary solution. You can't keep the chubby little boy locked up and punished forever. At some point, he reemerges. In the end, when I repressed him, I was only repressing myself.

Imagine all the effort and energy it takes to keep a portion of you locked away deep inside you so it doesn't stick its nose into your business. I could have focused all that energy into something positive, but I didn't realize it back then. With the help of a psychologist, I even made a physical representation of the emotional weight I'd been trying to control at all costs.

During one session, a psychologist asked me to draw something that represented everything I hated about my inner chubby boy. I grabbed a pencil and paper and the first thing that came to my mind was a cockroach. That's what I drew. I drew an S over it because the roach tried to suppress all my dreams and it was something I had to control at all costs. I left that session picturing the inner me as a cockroach. How horrible to imagine a cockroach living inside me! But back then, I didn't picture it like that. I clung to that image and even drew the letter S all around me to remind me of the cockroach I needed to control. I put an S on my car, on the side of my television, on my phone, on my computer. The idea was to never lose sight of him so that I could remember to repress him.

When my guide, Alicia, heard this story, she remained silent and then asked me a question. "Where does you inner chubby boy live?" she asked. I told her I felt like he lived in my heart. "Do you realize," she said, "that you're telling me that deep inside you lives . . . a cockroach?" My blood ran cold. I had never looked it at that way. We'd hit upon something big. I didn't want a cockroach living in my heart! A cockroach can carry all manner of disease and sicknesses. They say our nightmares tell of our greatest fears; they are a reflection of our daily worries. Dreaming of roaches means you need to make drastic changes in your life. I don't want these feelings inside my heart. I want to be happy every day, feeling satisfied and grateful for everything in my life.

When I realized all this, I could finally work on my inner chubby child the way I hope you will, too: with love, acceptance, and forgiveness. I learned that instead of treating that part of me with panic, anger, and rancor, I needed to take care of him, protect him, love him. Now, whenever he steps out of line, instead of punishing him, I take him by the hand and show him the right way. I tell him that together we can succeed. I've stopped punishing the little boy and all the emotions he represents, replacing them with love, forgiveness, and education.

It was time to choose something else to represent what was inside me. That roach inside my heart that represented pain now had to be replaced by something that stood for light and hope. The first thing that came to my mind was a star.

I've always loved the stars, from the time I used to climb onto the roof of my house and watch the stars in the night sky. Standing before the immense dark sky, I liked to imagine how people far, far away from my little town lived. I used to think, "Are the stars as bright in the United States as they are in my beautiful Venezuela?" I could spend hours lost in those thoughts. Even today, I love going to the beach at night and looking at the stars.

And that's how I changed that cockroach into a star. Stars

represent dreams, hopes, brilliance, prosperity, rebirth, everything positive. This is what I've wanted to feel every day of my life. By transforming the cockroach into a star, I knew that not only would I be filled with light, but every time someone discovered the chubby little boy inside me, they too would feel that light shine upon them. With tears in his eyes, the little boy inside me found his smile and his radiance again. I'd never tried seeing the chubby boy inside me—whom I'd tried to conceal out of shame for years—as a lamp that could illuminate me and those around me. It was one of the greatest changes of perspectives I've ever experienced.

To achieve this change, I started with forgiveness. I forgave him and forgave myself for all the times he had ruined a relationship or a new job or an opportunity. I forgave him for all the anger and frustration he had caused me. As I forgave myself, I started to make peace with all that had tormented me for so long. I learned to let go of the anger I felt for him and replaced it with acceptance, love, and gratefulness. I thanked him because if not for him, I wouldn't be where I am today. That chubby little boy is now the star of my heart. That little boy is my champion. Thanks to him and his story, I can now help, motivate, and transform the lives of millions of others around the world. Thanks to him, I know my purpose and passion, to illuminate the lives of my fellow Latinos and say Yes You Can!

After this transformation, that smiling little boy is now the one who yells out to remind me that our mission is to illuminate the lives of others, to help them find joy, love, health, and happiness. Now, he and I are one. My past is fused with my present so I can achieve the future.

Now that I'm thirty-four, I realize I have spent so many years invested in achieving this freedom, this emotional peace I feel today. And I could never have arrived here without the 7 essential steps we've explored in this book. First, I made a commitment to myself. Then I identified my emotional weight. I learned to set my goals. I created visualizations and many vision boards. I took action and made new, lasting habits to replace my old ones. And finally, I learned the importance of living in the present. After going through each of these phases and giving myself the necessary time to understand them, digest them, and put them into action in my life, I was finally able to unblock my emotions and truly be free and merge with the chubby little boy inside me. I forgave him, accepted him, loved him. And I used his inner glow to illuminate our way.

Today I accept the little boy inside me, I applaud him, value him, and thank him. Today I understand his purpose in my life. It's you, my little friend, who reminds me where I come from, where I am, and where I'm going. I went from asking, "Why did you ruin my life, little boy?" to saying "Thank you for everything you've taught me. Thank you for being part of my life and for being my gift from God."

I hope this book, these 7 steps, my story, and all the life lessons I've learned and shared here will help you alleviate your emotions, reduce your emotional weight, heal your soul, and transform the chubby little boy or girl inside you. This is the path toward peace, liberty, and happiness both inside and out. It's within you. It's in your hands. You have the light inside you. You only have to decide to discover it. I will always be here to support you, to inspire you to find your own brilliance and allow it to illuminate your path. YOU DESERVE IT! Yes You Can!

Put It into Practice!

TRANSFORM YOUR DARKNESS INTO LIGHT

It's your turn. From now on I want you to transform the darkness you've been carrying around inside you into light to illuminate your path. Take your chubby inner voice by the hand and take these 7 steps together.

1. On a piece of paper, draw what you think represents the chubby little boy or girl inside you, that image you've carried around with you all these years. Set aside the piece of paper and continue on to the next steps.
2. Accept yourself. Accept the chubby boy or girl inside you. Stop rejecting and punishing him or her. He/she is an essential part of your life and it's time to open the door, look at him/her, and say, "You are no longer my enemy. I'm no longer afraid."
3. Forgive yourself. Stop blaming the chubby child inside you for all that has gone wrong in your life. Embrace him/her. Forgive him/her. Forgive him/her for the anger, frustration, and sadness that he/she may have caused you in the past.
4. Make peace. Now that you have accepted and forgiven the injured child inside you, make peace with that part of yourself. Tell him or her, "You are no longer going to control me. We are now one and we are traveling the same path. I will change your name. You are now the light that will illuminate my life." Let go of that hurtful past to make room for a more glorious present.
5. Thank yourself. Thank the child inside you, because if it weren't for that child and for all you

have lived through together, you wouldn't be here today, bettering your life and refocusing on your dreams and your happiness.

6. Love yourself. The time has come to love that little child inside you. Fill your soul with deep affection and transform the darkness inside you into the light that can bring you so much joy.
7. Now take the paper again and write a new name or draw a new image of the chubby child inside you—something that represents your new love, forgiveness, peace, and acceptance for that being of light inside you. I changed my cockroach into a star. Make sure that the new image fills you with light and love. That's what you really deserve.

(TWELVE)

Balance Your Body, Mind, and Soul

THIS JOURNEY OF 7 steps we've taken to help you lose your emotional weight has been incredible. I know that after reading these pages, you're well on your way toward transforming yourself in the ways you truly deserve. With these tools, you've been learning to refocus your mind and spirit on what you want the most, on what is good for you. You're on the right track. Now, the time has come to refocus your body, that vessel taking you through life and toward your dreams. You've worked so hard on the inside; now it's time to work on the outside—for your health and for your general well-being. It's time to align your mind, body, and spirit.

I know you're wondering, "Where do I begin?" Obviously, you have to settle on a diet and exercise plan. But you can start detoxifying your body today with these five bits of advice.

1. CLEAN OUT YOUR PANTRY

Before you can clean out your body, first you have to clean out your pantry, the place where you head right to when hunger or anxiety strikes. Take the time to get rid of every temptation. If you leave the chocolate chip cookies and potato chips in there, aren't you going to eat them? Of course you are! It's like they're calling your name. So get rid of them. Toss all the processed food and the sugary snacks, and replace them with healthy items. That way, when you get a hankering for food, you'll only have healthy foods on hand and therefore there's a better chance you'll eat healthfully. Here's a list of food that is not only healthy but, when consumed as part of a portion-controlled diet, can also help you lose weight:

- *Healthy fats:* Not all fat is bad. There are several oils on the market that are better alternatives when it comes to cooking, as well as items with healthy oils that help our diets:
    - Canola, corn, olive, and soy oils
    - Avocado
    - Almond or peanut butter
    - Low-fat cottage cheese

- *Proteins:* Proteins are very important when we're on a diet, so always make sure to have some on hand. These include:
    - Red meat
    - Egg whites
    - Seafood
    - Turkey
    - Fish
    - Chicken

- *Carbohydrates:* A lot of diets eliminate carbohydrates, or carbs, from their plan. But did you know that carbohydrates help your body produce serotonin, a neurotransmitter that affects your well-being and helps you feel good inside? The goal is to select good carbs and knowing that the best time to eat them is at breakfast or lunch to give your body time to convert them into energy. The best sources of carbohydrates are as follows:
    - Oven-baked *arepas*
    - Rice, whole grain bread, and whole grain pasta
    - Oatmeal

  - Potatoes (and *boniato* and *malanga*)
  - Beans, lentils, and garbanzos
  - Fruits
  - Corn
  - Roasted or steamed yucca

- *Drinks:* There's nothing more crucial than drinking enough water. You should always have a bottle or pitcher handy. It's the best way to stay hydrated. If you're looking to supplement water with another beverage, avoid those that are filled with sugar and instead check out some of these:
  - Homemade lemonade (without sugar)
  - Coffee
  - Fruit teas (again, sugar free)
  - Green tea
  - Hibiscus tea

- *Desserts:* As part of the Yes You Can! diet, we've designed healthy dessert recipes to satiate that craving for something sweet. Besides these recipes, here are some other ideas:
  - Graham crackers
  - Sugar-free gelatin
  - Sugar-free gum
  - Fat-free, sugar-free yogurt

2. DETOX YOUR BODY

Whether you've broken your diet or are starting anew, these ingredients below will help you detox, that is, to get rid of the things your body doesn't need. Following these guidelines and including these items in your daily routine over the course of a week will help you get back on track to eating healthy or help you get started on your diet.

- *Water:* Water helps increase your blood's ability to carry oxygen so it becomes better at keeping your skin hydrated. Drinking water helps flush those toxins out of your body in your urine. So for your detox week, I recommend you drink a gallon of water every day.
- *Artichokes:* Not only are artichokes delicious, they are high in antioxidants and even help regulate your liver function. They help clean your system because they have two kinds of phytonutrients—cinarina and silymarin—which help the liver produce more bile to aid in the digestion of fat and in eliminating toxins. They also acts as a diuretic and regenerates liver cells.
- *Oatmeal:* Oatmeal is packed with a lot of fiber that helps us reactivate our digestive system and expel toxins from our bodies. Ideally, it's best to have plain oatmeal at breakfast, without any sweeteners or fruit mixed in.
- *Lemon:* Thanks to it's high vitamin C content, lemons, especially in water, help break down toxins and flush them from your system quickly. Add lemon to your water and include it in your meals.
- *Freshwater fish:* Freshwater fish such as salmon and sardines contain healthy fats and omega-3 acids, which reduce inflammation and optimize your immune system, helping your body remain free of toxins. Plus, the healthy fats act as a lubricant for your intestines, aiding in digestion.
- *Green tea:* This drink helps you burn calories, gives you energy, helps clean out your body, and regulates your digestive functions. So make green tea required drinking during your detox week. Drink two cups of green tea a day, hot or cold, without sugar. Try not to drink it too late in the day or in the evening or it might cause insomnia.
- *Raw vegetables:* Incorporating raw vegetables into your diet is the best way to infuse your body with the neces-

sary fiber and to hydrate it. It's important to include them in all your meals, so you can get all the vitamins, minerals, and antioxidants your body needs.

3. MOVE

No matter where you are, find a way to move and increase your heart rate. You don't have to live at the gym or be addicted to exercise. Regardless of whether you're at the office, at home, waiting for a bus, or wherever, you can always do something for your body. You can sweat out a lot of toxins, so I recommend you find a way to move: dance, work in the yard, take the stairs, go for a walk or a swim or a bike ride. Exercise! Do it at least three times a week for at least thirty-five minutes a day.

4. PLAN YOUR MEALS

Now that you have a list of healthy foods, the key is to plan out your meals. This is a pivotal step because if you don't plan out your menu for the week, it's easy to fall for the temptation of eating something that's not part of your diet. Planning your meals also helps you stay focused when you go grocery shopping. If you stick to your list, there's a better chance you won't buy any processed food that could do you more harm than good. On page 232, you can find a sample menu for your day. Use it as inspiration and motivation to continue on this healthy journey.

5. PRACTICE THE 7 STEPS TO REDUCE YOUR EMOTIONAL WEIGHT

While you incorporate this advice into your life, don't forget to continue working on the 7 steps to reduce your emotional weight. Remember that mind, body, and spirit go hand in hand. You shouldn't focus on one part while ignoring the others. So while you detox and learn to eat healthier, keep working on the 7 steps:

- Commit to yourself.
- Identify the problems in your path and get rid of them.
- Define your goals, revise them, and when you achieve them, set new ones.
- Continue making and repeating your affirmations according to each phase in your life.
- Use your vision board and update it depending on where you are in your life.
- Keep taking action and maintaining lasting, healthy habits.
- Focus on the amazing present, today, this gift from God.

SAMPLE MENU

Now, I want to leave you with a little gift: a preview of my next book. Yes, as you read the last pages of this book, I'm putting all my love and inspiration into my next project: a cookbook to help you lose weight with delicious Latin food that is certain to delight your palate. Here is a list of recipes that will keep you full throughout the day. Use them for inspiration to refocus on your diet and to stay on track toward the physical, mental, and emotional health you deserve. Thank you for joining me on this journey. We'll see each other in the next book. Yes You Can!

BREAKFAST

Protein Waffles

1 serving

½ cup oatmeal flour
1 Yes You Can! protein shake, Choco-Brownie flavor
1 egg
3 egg whites
1 teaspoon baking powder
1 tablespoon of flax seeds or chia seeds (optional)
1 teaspoon cocoa extract

1 pinch of cinnamon
Sugar-free chocolate syrup as garnish

1. Mix all the ingredients (except the chocolate syrup) together in a bowl.
2. Pour ⅓ of the mixture into a waffle iron and cook until golden brown.
3. Repeat the above step until you use all the mix.
4. Drizzle with sugar-free chocolate syrup, if you like.

SNACK

Stuffed Mushrooms

2 servings

1 small onion, diced
½ red pepper, diced
½ green pepper, diced
1 clove garlic, minced
4 medium-sized mushrooms
Cooking spray
6 ounces ground beef
½ tablespoon mustard
Salt and pepper, to taste
1 lemon

1. Preheat the oven to 350°F.
2. Clean all the vegetables well and remove the mushroom stems, leaving just the caps.
3. Spray a pan with the cooking spray. Over medium heat, cook the meat, onion, peppers, and garlic until the onion is translucent.
4. Pour the contents into a bowl, add the mustard and salt and pepper to taste, and mix together.
5. Spray a baking sheet with cooking spray. Fill the mushroom caps with the mixture, then place them meat-side-up on the baking sheet and bake for 15 to 20 minutes.

6. Remove from oven and allow to cool for 5 minutes.
7. Serve with a squeeze of lemon and enjoy.

LUNCH

Tostones with Beef

1 serving

Cooking spray
½ green plantain, peeled and cut into ½-inch round slices
3 ounces flank steak
Salt to taste
1 pinch of black pepper
1 bay leaf
1 large onion, diced small
½ red pepper, diced small
1 clove garlic, minced
¼ cup tomato puree
1 pinch of cumin

1. Preheat the oven to 350°F.
2. Spray a baking sheet with cooking spray. Place the plantain slices on it and bake for 30 minutes or until they are golden.
3. Remove the plantains from the oven. Squash each plantain slice with a plate, until they are flat.
4. Put the flattened slices back into the oven on a baking sheet and bake until they are golden brown, about 10 to 15 minutes.
5. Meanwhile, place the meat into a pot with salt to taste, the pepper, and bay leaf and fill with water to cover the meat. Cook it over medium heat for 20 minutes or until the meat is tender.
6. Throw away the bay leaf and drain the meat, reserving the broth. Pull or shred the beef.
7. Spray a pan with cooking spray and place over medium

heat. Add the onion, red pepper, and garlic. Sauté for 2 to 3 minutes.

8. Add the meat, tomato puree, cumin, and a bit of the reserved beef broth and stir well. Cook for 10 minutes over medium heat.
9. Plate the plantains and salt to taste. Pile meat on top of each one and drizzle with some of the reserved beef broth. Enjoy!

SWEET SNACK

Vanilla Flan

1 serving

1 cup water
1 unflavored gelatin packet
1 Yes You Can! protein shake, Vanilla flavor
2 packets artificial sweetener
Cinnamon to taste

1. Boil the water and pour into a bowl. Dissolve the gelatin in the water.
2. Add the Yes You Can! protein powder, the sweetener, and half a cup of cold water, and stir well.
3. Pour the mix into a silicone mold.
4. Refrigerate for 20 minutes and pop out of the mold onto a plate.
5. Add cinnamon to taste.

DINNER

Grouper Ceviche

6 servings

2 pounds grouper, skin and bones removed
Salt and pepper to taste
Juice of 6 limes
1 onion, diced
1 red pepper, cut into strips

1 handful of fresh cilantro, chopped
6 lettuce leaves for serving
Apple cider vinegar to taste

1. First cut the fish into strips, then into smaller cubes, and place into a large bowl.
2. Season the fish with salt and pepper and cover completely with lime juice.
3. Add the onion, red pepper, and cilantro.
4. Cover the bowl and store in the refrigerator for at least one hour.
5. The lemon will "cook" the fish. If the grouper is no longer transparent, it is sufficiently cured.
6. Serve with lettuce leaves, a splash of vinegar, and salt and pepper to taste. Enjoy!

RECOMMENDED READING

The Alchemist, Paulo Coelho
Heal Your Body, Louise Hay
Secrets of the Millionaire Mind, T. Harv Eker
The Power of Now, Eckart Tolle
Aligned Thinking, Jim Steffen
The Four Agreements, Don Miguel Ruiz
The Secret, Rhonda Byrne

ACKNOWLEDGMENTS

Dear Lord, THANK YOU for guiding me, giving me the gift of being able to open my eyes each morning so that I can continue the mission with which you have charged me: to help inspire others to lead a happier and healthier life. Thank you for being present in every moment of my life.

Thank you to my family for their unconditional love.

Thank you to the wonderful Yes You Can! team for their daily commitment to guiding people toward an easy, happy, and healthy lifestyle.

Thank you to Johanna Castillo, vice president and executive editor at Atria Books, and to the entire team at Simon & Schuster for believing in this book and helping me make it a reality.

And thank you, the readers, for the family that life gave me—the great Yes You Can! family—for all your love and support, for joining this movement to improve your quality of life. Thank you for proving that everyone who wants to succeed, if they commit 100 percent and let their hearts guide them, they, too, can succeed. Remember: I believe in you! Yes You Can!